Female
Reproductive System

Clinical Anatomy and Physiology

Akmal El-Mazny

C<small>ONTENTS</small>

PAGE

− I<small>NTRODUCTION</small>   1

− O<small>VERVIEW</small>   2

− O<small>VARIES</small>   7

− H<small>ORMONAL</small> C<small>ONTROL</small>   10

− O<small>VARIAN</small> C<small>YCLE</small>   18

− O<small>OCYTE</small> D<small>EVELOPMENT</small>   24

− O<small>VARIAN</small> F<small>ACTORS OF</small> I<small>NFERTILITY</small>   29

− F<small>ALLOPIAN</small> T<small>UBES</small>   54

− F<small>ERTILIZATION</small>   57

− T<small>UBAL</small> F<small>ACTORS OF</small> I<small>NFERTILITY</small>   59

− U<small>TERUS</small>   75

− E<small>NDOMETRIAL</small> C<small>YCLE</small>   79

− I<small>MPLANTATION</small>   82

− E<small>MBRYO</small> D<small>EVELOPMENT</small>   85

− U<small>TERINE</small> F<small>ACTORS OF</small> I<small>NFERTILITY</small>   86

− C<small>ERVIX</small>   101

− C<small>APACITATION</small>   103

− C<small>ERVICAL</small> F<small>ACTORS OF</small> I<small>NFERTILITY</small>   104

− R<small>EFERENCES</small>   108

INTRODUCTION

The female reproductive system consists of the hypothalamic-pituitary unit, the ovaries, the reproductive tract, and the external genitalia.

The functions of the female reproductive system are to produce and deliver oocytes, for sexual reproduction, and produce hormones that regulate reproductive function and secondary sex characteristics.

Abnormalities in anatomic or physiologic function affect the development and delivery of gametes, and potential fertility.

Female factor infertility can be divided into several categories: ovarian, tubal and peritoneal, uterine, cervical, and other.

Management of female factors affecting fertility may include medical treatment, surgical intervention, or assisted reproductive techniques.

This book provides a comprehensive review of the clinical anatomy and physiology specific to female reproductive system, emphasizing causes and management of female infertility.

By developing a clear understanding of what is normal, you will better understand abnormalities affecting female fertility and the mechanisms behind treatment.

OVERVIEW

Basic Embryology

Sex determination takes place at the time of fertilization through the coupling of two gametes, either each with one X chromosome (XX in females) or such with an X and a Y chromosome (XY in males).

Primarily, the male (female) phenotype is determined by the presence (or absence) of the Y chromosome with its genes, even though genes on other chromosomes are also involved.

In addition to the genetic factors, hormonal regulation also plays an important role during the various developmental steps.

During the first 6 weeks the genital system is sex-indifferent and it is only then that the gonads as well as the internal and external genitalia form under hormonal influence.

In the male fetus, the supporting (Sertoli) cells of the testes form the antimüllerian hormone (AMH), which causes the paramesoneophric (Müllerian) duct to atrophy.

The development of female genitalia is characterized by atrophy of the mesonephric (Wolffian) duct and retention of the paramesoneophric (Müllerian) duct, out of which the fallopian tube, the uterus, and the upper part of the vagina arise.

The urogenital sinus forms the genital swellings, the urethral folds, the genital tubercle, and the external genitalia (lowest part of the vagina, vaginal vestibule, labia majora and minora as well as the clitoris).

In the ovarian cortex, the primordial germ cells are surrounded by the follicle cells that come from the coelomic epithelium and form the primordial follicles.

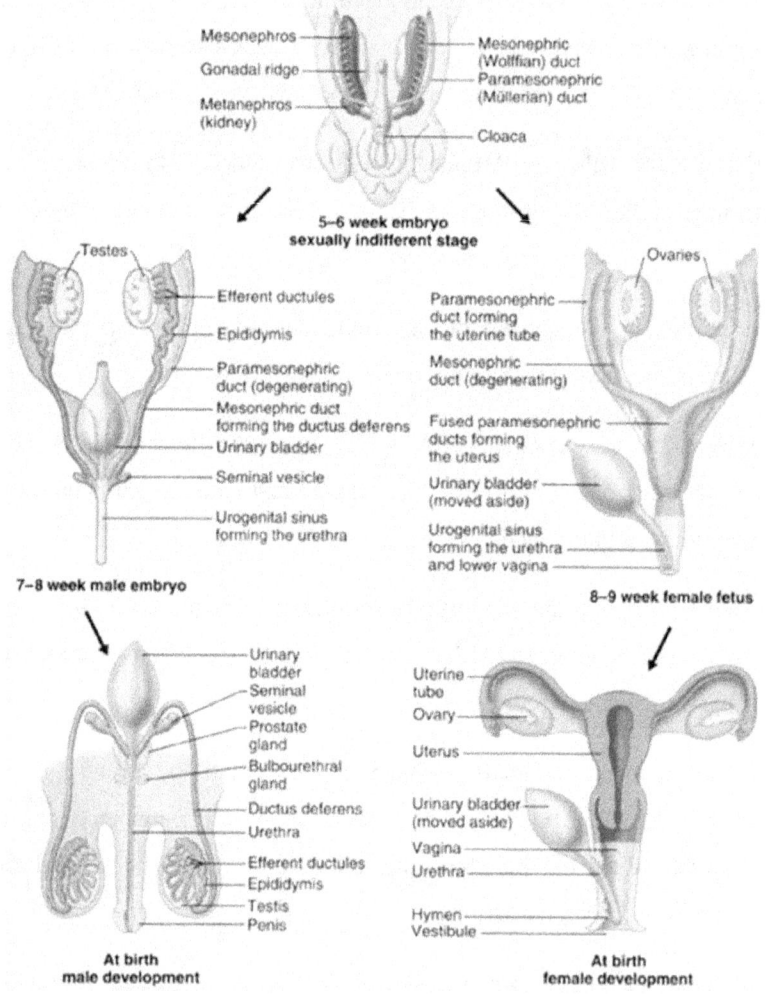

Sexual Differentation

Basic Anatomy and Physiology

The female reproductive system is a complicated but fascinating subject.

It has the capability to function intimately with nearly every other body system for the purpose of reproduction.

The female reproductive system consists of the hypothalamic-pituitary unit, the ovaries, the reproductive tract, and the external genitalia.

The functions of the female reproductive system are to produce and deliver oocytes, for sexual reproduction, and produce hormones that regulate reproductive function and secondary sex characteristics.

The female reproductive organs can be subdivided into the internal and external genitalia.

The internal genitalia are those organs that are within the true pelvis: the ovaries, fallopian tubes, uterus, cervix, and vagina.

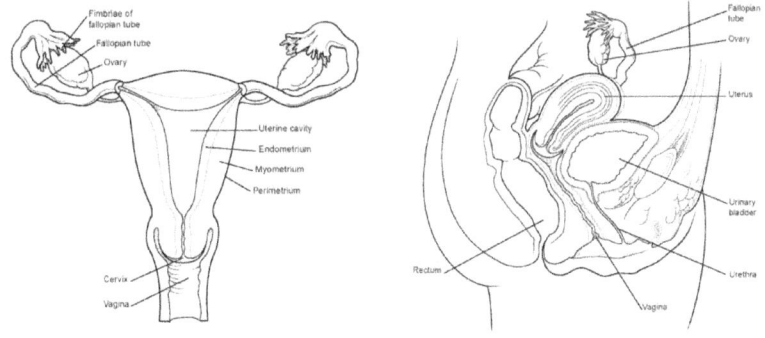

Female Reproductive System

The external genitalia lie outside the true pelvis: the perineum, mons pubis, clitoris, urethral (urinary) meatus, labia majora and minora, vestibule, greater vestibular (Bartholin) glands, Skene glands, and periurethral area.

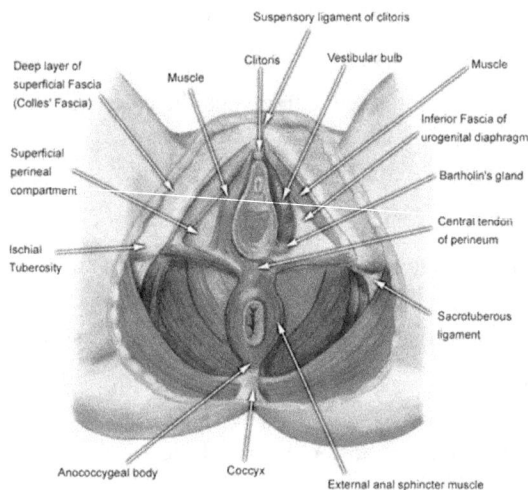

Deep Structures of Female External Genitalia

Female Infertility

Infertility is defined by the World Health Organization (WHO) as the absence of conception after at least 12 months of unprotected intercourse.

This condition affects approximately 10-15% of reproductive-aged couples.

Isolated conditions of the female are responsible for infertility in 35% of cases, isolated conditions of the male in 30%, conditions of both the male and female in 20%, and unexplained causes in 15%.

To understand the rationale for deciding what should be included in a female fertility evaluation, it is helpful to consider what is required in order to establish a normal pregnancy:

– The production of adequate spermatozoa.

– The release of a normal preovulatory oocyte.

– The normal transport of the gametes to the ampullary portion of the fallopian tube (where fertilization occurs).

– The subsequent transport of the cleaving embryo into the endometrial cavity for implantation and development.

Female factor infertility can be divided into several categories: ovarian, tubal and peritoneal, uterine, cervical, and other.

A basic evaluation for female infertility includes an assessment for ovulation, tubal patency, and normality of the uterine cavity.

Management of female factors affecting fertility may include medical treatment, surgical intervention, or assisted reproductive techniques.

OVARIES

The ovaries are paired organs located on either side of the uterus within the mesovarium portion of the broad ligament below the uterine tubes.

At birth, a female has approximately 1-2 million eggs, but only 300 of these eggs ever mature and are released for the purpose of fertilization.

The ovaries are small and oval-shaped, exhibit a grayish color, and have an uneven surface.

The actual size of an ovary depends on a woman's age and hormonal status; the ovaries are approximately 3-5 cm in length during childbearing years and become much smaller and atrophic once menopause occurs.

A cross-section of the ovary reveals many cystic structures that vary in size representing ovarian follicles at different stages of development and degeneration.

Several ligaments support the ovary:

– The ovarian ligament connects the uterus and ovary.

– The posterior portion of the broad ligament forms the mesovarium, which supports the ovary and houses the vascular supply.

– The suspensory (infundibular) ligament of the ovary, a peritoneal fold overlying the ovarian vessels, attaches the ovary to the pelvic side wall.

Blood supply to the ovary is via the ovarian artery; both right and left ovarian arteries originate directly from the descending aorta at the level of the L2 vertebra, and enter the ovary at the hilum.

The left ovarian vein drains into the left renal vein, and the right ovarian vein empties directly into the inferior vena cava.

Lymphatic drainage of the ovary is primarily to the lateral aortic nodes; however, the iliac nodes may also be involved.

Nerve supply to the ovaries, through the ovarian, hypogastric, and aortic plexuses, run with the vasculature within the suspensory ligament of the ovary entering the ovary at the hilum.

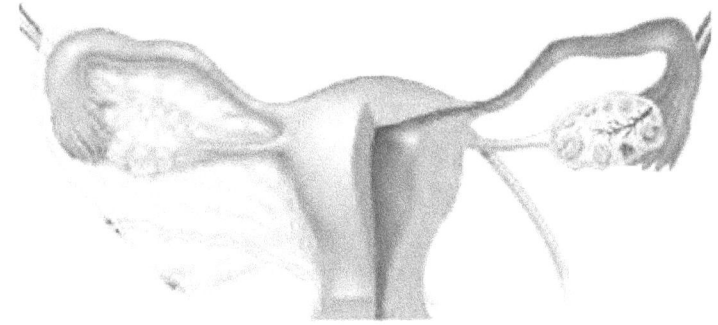

Gross Anatomy of the Ovaries

Microscopic Anatomy

The ovaries are covered externally by a layer of simple cuboidal epithelium called germinal (ovarian) epithelium.

Beneath this layer is a dense connective tissue capsule, the tunica albuginea.

The main body of the ovary is divided into an outer cortex and an inner medulla.

– The cortex is dense and granular and contains numerous ovarian follicles in various stages of development.

– The medulla is loose connective tissue with abundant blood vessels, lymphatic vessels, and nerve fibers.

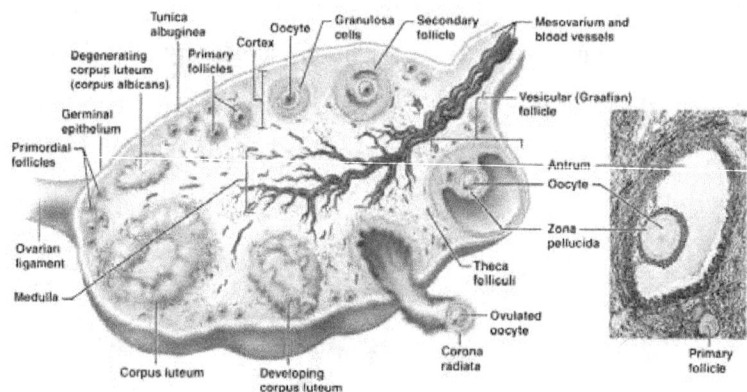

Microscopic Anatomy of the Ovary

Functional Anatomy

– The ovary cyclically produces gametes; the number of oocytes (germ cells) available is determined during fetal development and continues to decline by either ovulation or atresia until menopause occurs.

– It also cyclically secretes hormones (androgens, estrogens, progestins) that prepare the reproductive tract for oocyte transport, fertilization, implantation and pregnancy, and it controls the hypothalamic-pituitary unit through negative and positive feedback mechanisms.

HORMONAL CONTROL

There are four major functional compartments involved in reproduction, each has a specific function: the hypothalamus, the pituitary gland and the ovaries, which compose the hypothalamic-pituitary-ovarian (HPO) axis; and the hormonally-responsive functional endometrium lining the uterus.

In the presence of low levels of estrogen, the arcuate nucleus of the hypothalamus releases gonadotropin-releasing hormone.

This hormone signals the anterior pituitary to produce the gonadotropins LH and FSH.

These gonadotropins in turn induce the development and maturation of ovarian follicles that contain the actual oocytes.

During the growth process, the follicles produce increased amounts of estradiol.

This increase in estrogen production develops the endometrium and thins the increasing amounts of cervical mucus.

When the estradiol level reaches an appropriate level, generally when the follicle is mature, the pituitary releases a large amount of LH.

LH surge causes the final maturation of the oocyte and stimulates the event of ovulation.

After the oocyte is released, that is, ovulation occurs, the sac containing the oocyte undergoes metamorphosis with growth of new blood vessels and becomes a functioning gland called the corpus luteum.

The corpus luteum produces progesterone in large amounts and estrogen in smaller amounts.

Progesterone stabilizes the endometrium and thickens the cervical mucus.

The lifespan of corpus luteum is about 14 days, unless pregnancy occurs.

If the woman does not conceive in a particular cycle, after 14 days, the corpus luteum stops producing progesterone, the endometrium is no longer stable, and menses begin.

The normal menstrual cycle length is 25 to 35 days; this cyclicity is determined by changing sensitivities of the hypothalamic-pituitary unit to estrogens and progestins.

The HPO axis also involves a negative feedback loop in which gonadal secretions produced in response to pituitary gonadotropins inhibit further secretion of gonadotropins.

The HPO axis in the female also involves a positive feedback loop in which ovarian estrogen produced in response to pituitary FSH enhances pituitary secretion of LH and FSH.

Functional Compartment	Location	Hormone or Function
- Hypothalamus	- Arcuate nucleus	- GnRH
- Anterior pituitary	- Gonadotropin	- FSH
		- LH
- Ovary	- Follicle	- Estradiol
	- Corpus luteum	- Progesterone
		- Inhibin
		- Activin
		- Anti-Mullerian hormone
- Uterus	- Endometrium	- Proliferative
		- Secretory
		- Menses

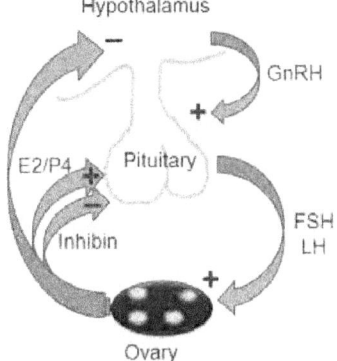

Hypothalamic-Pituitary-Ovarian (HPO) Axis

Hypothalamus - GnRH

GnRH is synthesized and secreted by neurons in the arcuate nucleus of the hypothalamus and diffuses into the hypothalamic-hypophyseal portal vessels, which transport it to the anterior pituitary gland.

Through pulsatile release, GnRH stimulates the gonadotropes to produce FSH and LH.

The activity of this decapeptide can be modified by changing one or more amino acids; this creates GnRH agonists or antagonists that are often used as adjuncts to infertility and other medical disorders.

Anterior Pituitary - FSH

FSH is a heterodimeric glycoprotein synthesized in gonadotropes in the anterior pituitary.

It has a relatively long half-life in the plasma, normally 3-4 hours; peripheral plasma levels of FSH do not reflect pulsatile GnRH secretion.

FSH stimulates granulosa cells of the ovarian follicle and the luteinized cells of the corpus luteum.

It is considered the critical regulator of follicular development because it is capable of stimulating follicular development by itself.

FSH is suppressed by rising estradiol from the growing follicle; cyclic levels are at their maximum on Day 3 and midcycle surge.

The number of primary follicles which begin to enlarge and respond to FSH is related to the age and total number of oocytes present in the ovary.

Since there is no maturing follicle to suppress FSH, during menopause, FSH is elevated.

Anterior Pituitary - LH

LH is a heterodimeric glycoprotein synthesized in the same gonadotropes in the anterior pituitary as FSH.

LH has a shorter plasma half life (about 20 minutes) than FSH, so peripheral plasma levels do reflect the pronounced pulsatile pattern of GnRH secretion.

LH is secreted in a pulsatile manner:

– In the follicular phase, the pulse interval is normally 90 min.

– In the luteal phase it is about 2 to 3 hours.

LH stimulates mature granulosa cells of the preovulatory follicle and their successor cells, the luteinized cells of the corpus luteum.

LH is capable of maintaining the lifespan of the corpus luteum beyond the normal luteal phase of the menstrual cycle; however, LH is rapidly degraded when administered by injection.

HCG mimics LH, and can therefore stimulate ovulation and support the luteal phase; hCG has a much longer half life and is slower to degrade when administered by injection.

LH has the following stimulatory effects on ovarian cells:

– Increases availability of free cholesterol.

– Stimulates production of androgens in ovarian theca and interstitial cells by increasing enzymes for androgen biosynthesis.

– Increases production of progesterone and estradiol in the corpus luteum.

– Increases plasminogen activator synthesis and secretion in granulosa cells of the preovulatory follicle.

– Stimulates resumption of meiosis in the oocyte at midcycle.

Ovary - Sex Steroids

Although the ovary secretes many substances steroid hormones including androgens, estrogens and progestins, appear to be among the most important.

Androgens are synthesized in the theca and interstitial cells and are important as substrates for estrogen biosynthesis.

The adrenal glands are the principal source of circulating androgens (dehydroepiandrosterone, androstenedione, and testosterone) in women.

The increase in synthesis of adrenal androgens at puberty (called adrenarche) stimulates the development of axillary, pubic and facial hair.

High levels of androgens suppress progesterone synthesis in granulosa cells.

Although the ovaries and adrenals produce similar quantities of androstenedione and testosterone, most of the ovarian androgens are converted to estrogens in the ovaries and in peripheral tissues.

Most of the testosterone in the plasma of the adult female is formed by peripheral conversion of androstenedione by peripheral 17β-hydroxysteroid dehydrogenase.

Estradiol is considered the most important product of the granulosa cells of the developing follicle; estrone is a less active estrogen than estradiol.

Estradiol concentrations in plasma reach a peak during the late follicular phase, decline after ovulation and then rise again during the luteal phase.

Progesterone is considered the most important product of the corpus luteum.

Ovary - Inhibins and Activins

Inhibin is a heterodimeric glycoprotein consisting of an alpha and a beta subunit and is synthesized by granulosa and luteal cells of the ovary.

FSH stimulates granulosa cells to synthesize and secrete inhibin, so that as follicles enlarge, they produce increasing amounts of the hormone.

Inhibin preferentially inhibits synthesis and secretion of FSH but not LH by pituitary gonadotropes (negative feedback).

Inhibin production is low at the beginning of the menstrual cycle, then increases late in the follicular phase and reaches a peak prior to the preovulatory surge of FSH and LH.

After ovulation, inhibin levels decrease slightly, followed by a final rise in the midluteal phase to a level twice that at midcycle.

As the corpus luteum regresses, inhibin levels decline and FSH levels rise with the beginning of the next menstrual cycle.

The ovarian granulosa cells also secrete activin, a dimeric protein consisting of two of the β subunits of inhibin.

Activin amplifies the effect of FSH on granulosa cells in the ovary and also increases the synthesis of the FSH β subunit in the anterior pituitary.

Neuroendocrine Control

− Inhibin, acts on the pituitary to suppress the synthesis and release of FSH, but does not impact LH.

− In the follicular phase, estrogen exerts negative feedback by decreasing the pulse amplitude thereby decreasing FSH and LH pulse amplitude.

− In the luteal phase, progesterone and testosterone decrease GnRH pulse frequency resulting in decreased FSH and LH pulse frequency.

− Testosterone inhibits gonadotropin gene expression in the anterior pituitary; women with elevated serum testosterone levels often do not have normal menstrual cycles.

− GnRH is also inhibited by high concentrations of prolactin; breastfeeding may act as a contraceptive.

– The thyroid can also impact the HPO axis; thyrotropin-releasing hormone (TRH) at high concentrations stimulates the pituitary gland to produce prolactin; patients with hypothyroidism or secondary hyperthyroidism also have decreased gonadotropin secretion.

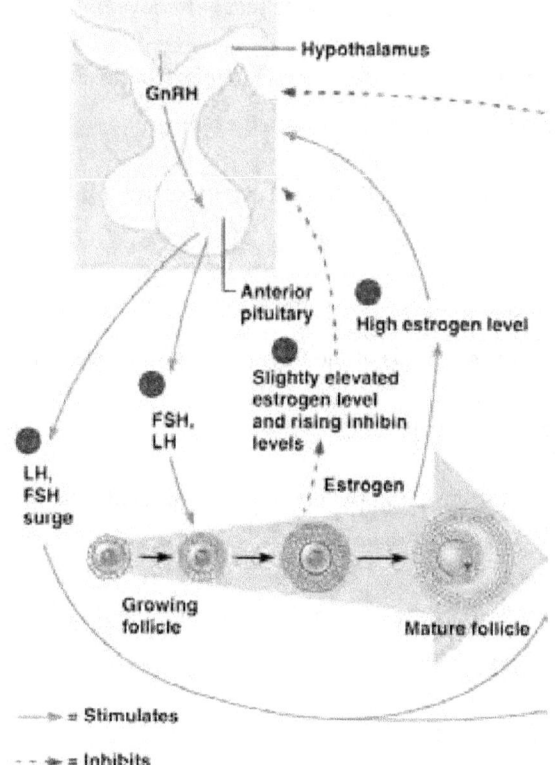

Neuroendocrine Control

OVARIAN CYCLE

The follicle is the basic functional unit of the ovary.

Each follicle consists of an oocyte surrounded by one or more layers of specialized cells (granulosa, theca) which secrete autocrine, paracrine, and endocrine factors.

The follicle grows under the influence of gonadotropins (FSH, LH) and intraovarian regulators (estradiol, IGF-I, activin).

Development from a primordial follicle to a preovulatory follicle takes three to four menstrual cycles.

Follicular Phase

Primordial Follicle

– Primordial follicles are formed during fetal life and are not believed to require gonadotropins for formation; however, females lacking functional FSH receptors have poorly developed ovaries.

– A primordial follicle consists of an oocyte and a single layer of epithelial cells.

– The oocyte is arrested in the first meiotic prophase.

– During the first cycle of development the oocyte grows to about 100 microns in diameter and the epithelial cells enlarge and become cuboidal granulosa cells; at this point, the oocyte is referred to as the "primary follicle".

−FSH receptors are first detectable on the plasma membrane of granulosa cells.

−The granulosa cells respond to FSH by proliferating faster.

Preantral Follicle

−During the first to second cycles of development, the primary follicle progresses to the preantral stage.

−Oocyte meiosis remains arrested.

−The oocyte completes the first step of meiotic maturation, which includes germinal vesicle breakdown and metaphase I after the mid-cycle LH surge.

−Preantral follicles respond to the midcycle surge of FSH during the second to third cycles of development by growing rapidly; this event is called recruitment.

−All recruited follicles produce sex steroid hormones in amounts proportional to their size and degree of maturation.

−A single follicle, the most mature follicle, becomes dominant.

−The remaining follicles degenerate through a process called atresia.

−The emergence of the single dominant follicle appears to result from the inhibin-induced decline in plasma FSH concentrations.

−Once a dominant follicle is selected, rising serum hormone levels of inhibin and estradiol suppress FSH.

− Local production of estradiol by the dominant follicle amplifies the response to FSH.

− Estradiol synthesis continues to increase exponentially in response to FSH.

Antral Follicle

− Fluid accumulates among the granulosa cells forming a fluid-filled cavity, the antrum.

− After the antrum is formed, the follicle is termed a "secondary follicle".

Preovulatory Follicle

− During the last cycle of development (third or fourth cycle), the dominant follicle attains its maximal size and the theca layer vascularizes; this represents the "Graafian follicle".

− The oocyte (meiosis still arrested) has the capacity to proceed to metaphase II and complete meiotic maturation after fertilization.

− Granulosa cells of immature follicles have few LH receptors so they don't respond to LH at physiological LH concentrations.

− The theca cells (and the interstitial cells) do have LH receptors and they respond to LH.

− One of the actions of FSH on granulosa cells during the follicular phase of the menstrual cycle is to induce LH receptors so that granulosa cells of the preovulatory Graafian follicle become responsive to LH as well as to FSH.

– After the LH/FSH surge prior to ovulation, the granulosa cells initially decrease their LH and FSH receptors and then increase them as the granulosa cells luteinize to become the corpus luteum.

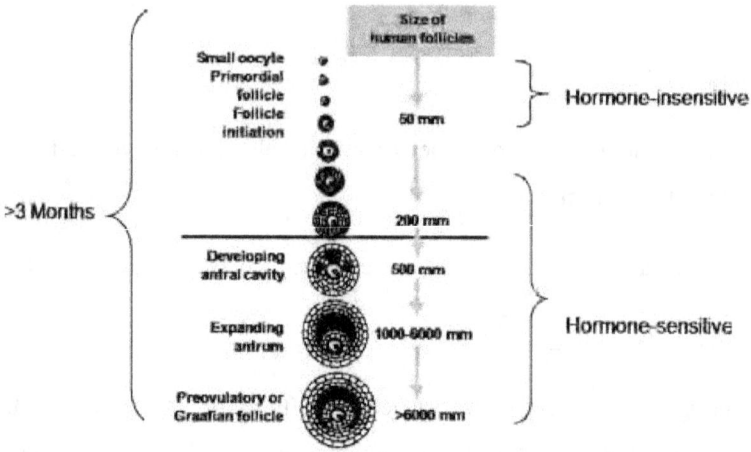

Follicle Development

Ovulation Phase

– LH triggers several processes that culminate in ovulation.

– LH causes a resumption of oocyte meiosis, and metaphase I is completed.

– The first polar body is extruded, and meiosis then halts in metaphase II.

– An increase in follicular pressure, combined with LH-activated breakdown of the follicular wall results in follicular rupture.

– The cumulus-oocyte complex is ovulated 34-36 hours after the onset of the LH surge, and the remaining granulosa and theca cells luteinize.

Luteal Phase

– After ovulation the follicular cells luteinize and form the corpus luteum (literally, yellow body).

– They acquire the capacity to secrete progesterone, and lipid droplets accumulate in the cells.

– If the oocyte is fertilized and implants in the endometrium, the corpus luteum remains active and secretes progesterone in large amounts and estradiol in smaller amounts.

– Progesterone from the corpus luteum prepares the endometrium for implantation and maintains the fetal-placental unit during the first half of the first trimester of pregnancy.

– The corpus luteum requires low levels of LH for continued function.

– LH stimulates the production of progesterone and estradiol, and FSH stimulates the production of estradiol only.

– If fertilization and implantation do not occur, the corpus luteum degenerates (called luteolysis), and progesterone declines within 10 days after ovulation.

– Unlike the variable length of the follicular phase of the menstrual cycle, the luteal phase has a lifespan of about 14 days; this lifespan is due to the fairly consistent lifespan of the corpus luteum.

– However, if pregnancy occurs, the corpus luteum is rescued by hCG that is produced by the implanted trophoblasts.

−LH and hCG are similar in structure; hCG may be thought of as long acting LH.

−In clinical situations hCG injections are used to act like LH, particularly to induce ovulation or stimulate luteal progesterone production.

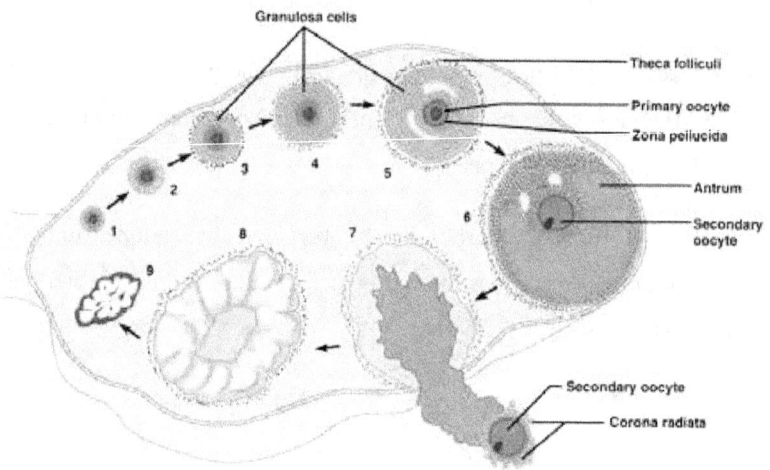

Ovarian Cycle

OOCYTE DEVELOPMENT

The ovaries and germ cells (which develop into oocytes) form during the first few weeks of embryonic life.

These germ cells rapidly divide by a process called mitosis, in which each new daughter cell contains the same number of chromosomes as the parent cell.

During the first trimester of embryonic growth, these preoocyte cells are called oogonium (plural: oogonia).

During the second trimester of life, the 46 chromosomes start to replicate through the process of meiosis but remain within the cell.

At this stage of meiosis, the cell is called a primary oocyte (primitive ovum not yet fully developed).

At this point, further chromosome separation and oocyte development are arrested until after puberty.

These primary oocytes are surrounded by a layer of epithelium that gives rise to the primordial follicles.

About 1700 germ cells are present before migration to the genital ridge begins.

However, these multiply during the process of migration, reaching a peak of 7 million oocytes at midgestation.

The primordial germ cells increase in size early in their development and become oogonia.

At midgestation, they begin the first meiotic division, becoming primary oocytes.

This prophase lasts until just before ovulation, which may occur 12 to 40 or more years later.

In this state, they are no longer capable of multiplication and, in fact, steadily decline in number.

About 400 ova are released through the process of ovulation during a woman's lifetime.

The remaining ova undergo atresia (a normal process affecting the primordial ovarian follicles in which death of the ovum results in degeneration) so that, by the time of the menopause, few are present.

The oocyte remains in this stage until it is either eliminated by atresia or succeeds in reaching the maturation stage and resumption of meiosis (reduction division) at the time of ovulation.

Meiosis has two purposes: reduction to the haploid number of chromosomes to one half of the normal, or 23, and recombination of genetic information.

The first meiotic division, which begins during fetal life, is completed prior to ovulation and produces a secondary oocyte containing 23 chromosomes and the first polar body containing 23 chromosomes, each with 2 daughter chromatids.

A polar body is composed of cell division products that result from meiosis.

The second meiotic division, which is initiated after ovulation, is completed at sperm penetration and produces a mature oocyte containing 23 chromosomes and a polar body containing 23 chromosomes, each with a single chromatid.

When the oocyte and sperm combine at fertilization, the full complement of 46 chromosomes is restored and a new life is created.

The second polar body will degenerate like the first.

As a result of the combined meiotic processes, a single mature oocyte is produced and 2 or 3 polar bodies degenerate.

This is in contrast to the meiotic process in males where a single precursor cell gives rise to 4 mature sperm.

Oocyte Maturation and Ovulation

– Resumption of meiosis begins within the ovarian follicle in response to the LH surge.

– The granulosa cells, that is, the cumulus oophorus, expands.

– The first polar body is extruded and the oocyte progresses into metaphase of the second meiotic division.

– Meiosis stops in metaphase II until fertilization.

Fertilization

Contractions of the oviductal muscles direct the oocyte into the ampulla of the fallopian tube where it remains for about 3 days while the ampullary-isthmic sphincter remains contracted.

The oocytes remain fertile for only 15-18 hours after ovulation while sperm are motile for 24 hours to several days after ejaculation.

When a sperm encounters the zona pellucida, it undergoes an acrosome reaction; this breaks down the acrosomal membrane.

The sperm head membrane binds to the sperm receptor, which is followed by fusion with the oolemma.

Microvilli on the oocyte surface surround the sperm head and the oocyte undergoes the cortical reaction (release of cortical granules).

The zona pellucida hardens and no other sperm can penetrate the oolemma.

The oocyte nucleus completes maturation to yield the female pronucleus and the second polar body; the sperm nucleus forms the male pronucleus.

The corona radiata is the layer of granulosa cells surrounding the oocyte; the zona pellucida is an extracellular layer of proteins surrounding the oocyte.

Egg Activation

The process of egg activation occurs after fertilization, and involves the completion of the second meiotic division and initiation of embryonic development.

Mitosis begins and there are changes in maternal messenger ribonucleic acids and protein synthesis.

Exocytosis of cortical granules blocks polyspermy and cytoskeletal rearrangement occurs.

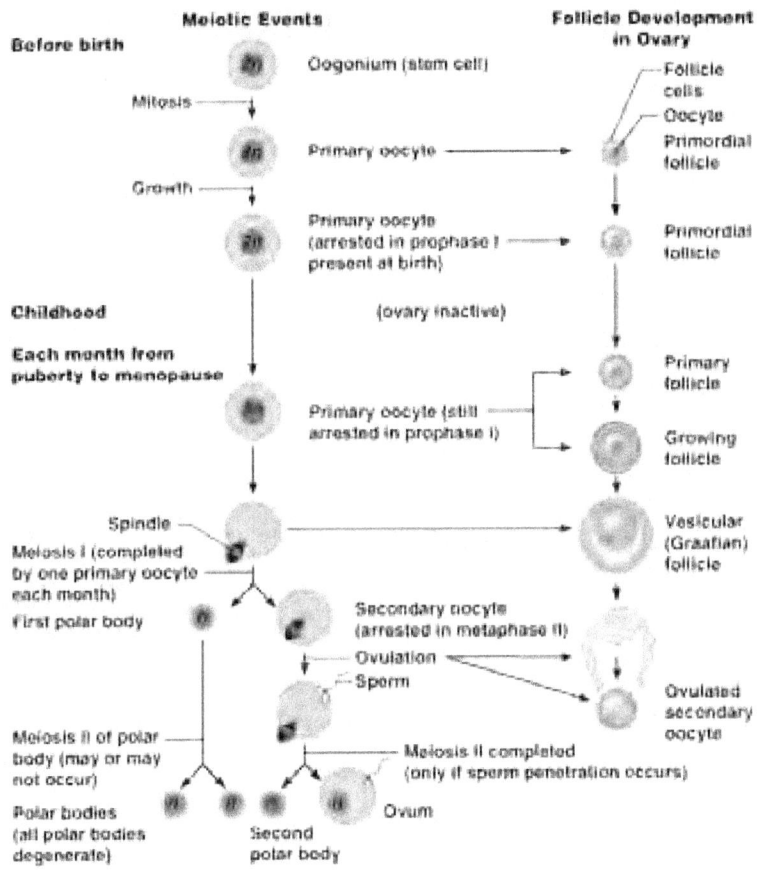

Oocyte Development

OVARIAN FACTORS OF INFERTILITY

Oogenesis occurs in the ovary from the first trimester of embryonic life and is completed by 28-30 weeks of gestation.

By then, approximately 7 million oocytes are present; they are arrested at the prophase stage of the first meiosis division.

Subsequently, the number of oocytes decreases because of a continuous process of atresia.

At birth, the pool of oocytes is reduced to approximately 2 million.

By menarche, approximately 500,000 oocytes are present.

Those oocytes are used throughout the reproductive years until menopause.

The ovulatory process is initiated once the hypothalamus-pituitary-ovarian axis matures and FSH and LH, under the regulation of GnRH, acquire their normal secretory patterns.

From the cohort of follicles available each month, only a single oocyte is selected, establishes dominance, and develops to the preovulatory stage.

During follicular development, the granulosa cells secrete increasing amounts of E_2, initially down-regulating the secretion of FSH.

Later, through a positive feedback mechanism, E_2 generates the LH surge that triggers the ovulatory process, induces the resumption of meiosis by the oocyte, and stimulates the formation of the corpus luteum and subsequent progesterone secretion.

Causes

Ovulatory dysfunction is defined as an alteration in the frequency and duration of the menstrual cycle.

Failure to ovulate is the most common infertility problem.

Absence of ovulation can be associated with primary amenorrhea, secondary amenorrhea, or oligomenorrhea.

Hypergonadotropic Hypogonadism

Hypergonadotropic hypogonadism is often related to gonadal development failure, as in Turner syndrome, where the karyotype 45,X indicates an absence of an X chromosome.

These patients present with sexual infantilism associated with short stature, webbed neck, and cubitus valgus.

Streak gonads replace their ovaries, but they have a small uterus and normal fallopian tubes and vagina.

This condition is associated with elevated FSH and LH and low estrogen.

Other chromosomal abnormalities include 46,XX, which is associated with partial deletions of the short or long arm of one of the X chromosomes, and mosaicism (eg, X/XXX; X/XX/XXX; pure gonadal dysgenesis; 46,XX; 46,XY).

Hypergonadotropic hypogonadism resulting in primary amenorrhea can also be seen in patients with a history of being treated with certain alkylating chemotherapy or pelvic radiation.

Chronic disease conditions, high levels of stress, and starvation or malnutrition are other possible etiologies.

Structural entities associated with primary amenorrhea include congenital absence of the uterus, vagina, or hymen (cryptomenorrhea).

Secondary amenorrhea is the absence of menses for more than 6 months in a woman who has previously menstruated.

In the absence of pregnancy, this condition is related to dysfunction of the endocrine system and can be related to thyroid, adrenal, and pituitary disorders, including tumors.

One common cause of secondary amenorrhea is premature ovarian failure, which is the loss of ovarian function by the age of 40.

Oligomenorrhea is a dysfunction of the hypothalamus-pituitary-ovarian axis and is the most common ovulatory disorder associated with infertility.

Patients with this disorder present with a history of irregular menstrual cycles that fluctuate from 35 days to 2-5 months, sometimes associated with a history of dysfunctional uterine bleeding or prolonged periods of breakthrough bleeding.

Patients may have symptoms of hyperandrogenism, acne, hirsutism, and baldness, obesity is frequently associated and aggravates the prognosis.

Although these patients are not sterile, their fertility is decreased, and the obstetrical outcome is generally poor because of an increased risk of pregnancy loss.

Hypogonadotropic Hypogonadism

Hypogonadotropic hypogonadism refers to suppression of GnRH pulsatility from the hypothalamus, resulting in lack of production of FSH and LH from the pituitary and lack of production of ovarian hormones.

Causes of hypogonadotropic hypogonadism include eating disorders, such as anorexia, bulimia, and disordered eating.

Extreme exercise, especially in combination with disordered eating, is also associated with hypothalamic suppression, as are hyperprolactinemia and hypothyroidism.

CNS lesions, such as craniopharyngioma, can lead to hypogonadotropic hypogonadism.

Kallmann syndrome is caused by failure of the GnRH neurons to migrate during fetal development and is associated with anosmia (inability to smell) and primary amenorrhea.

Hormonal assessment reveals FSH and LH in the low-normal range or very suppressed, less than 3 mIU/mL; estradiol is also suppressed to less than 30 pg/mL.

Longstanding hypogonadotropic hypogonadism is associated with low bone density due to prolonged hypoestrogenism.

Treatment is based on correcting the underlying pathology, treating eating disorders, central nervous system lesions, etc.

If hypogonadotropic hypogonadism persists, then treatment involves the use of gonadotropins to induce ovulation.

Polycystic Ovarian Syndrome (PCOS)

PCOS is the most common endocrinopathy in women.

It has been shown to occur in 4 to 6% of reproductive-aged women, though the prevalence has been reported to be as high as 10%.

It is also considered the single most common cause of infertility due to anovulation.

Prolactin Disorders

Prolactinomas are the most common pituitary adenoma, accounting for 40%.

Prolactinomas are considered microadenomas if the size is less than 10 mm, and macroadenomas if greater than 10 mm.

Macroadenomas can cause visual symptoms due to their size and compression of the optic chiasm.

Secretion of high levels of prolactin suppresses production of GnRH, leading to decreased FSH and LH, and hypoestrogenism.

Prolactinemia results in galactorrhea and suppresses gonadotropin secretion, leading to amenorrhea.

Presenting symptoms are, therefore, galactorrhea, amenorrhea or both.

Advanced Age

The prevalence of infertility rises dramatically as age increases, and also with marriage duration because of less frequent intercourse and/or the use of contraception.

Studies report that among Mormons, fertility appears to be stable until age 36 years, declines slightly until age 40 years, and is followed by a sharp decline after age 42 years.

Additionally, in the North American Hutterite population where contraception is condemned, infertility rates are 11% after age 34, 33% after at age 40 and 87% at age 45.

Chromosomal Abnormalities

Chromosomal abnormalities and poor oocyte quality are 2 examples of causes of poor embryonic quality, low implantation rate, increased miscarriage, and low birth rates.

Similar conclusions can be drawn from the experience of many IVF programs.

Gene	Encoded Protein	Effect of Deficiency
BMP15	Bone morphogenetic protein 15	Hypergonadotrophic ovarian failure (POF4)
BMPR1B	Bone morphogenetic protein receptor 1B	Ovarian dysfunction, hypergonadotrophic hypogonadism and acromesomelic chondrodysplasia
CBX2; M33	Chromobox protein homolog 2 ; Drosophila polycomb class	Autosomal 46,XY, male-to-female sex reversal
CHD7	Chromodomain-helicase-DNA-binding protein 7	CHARGE syndrome and Kallmann syndrome (KAL5)
DIAPH2	Diaphanous homolog 2	Hypergonadotrophic, premature ovarian failure (POF2A)
FGF8	Fibroblast growth factor 8	Normosmic hypogonadotrophic hypogonadism and Kallmann syndrome (KAL6)
FGFR1	Fibroblast growth factor receptor 1	Kallmann syndrome (KAL2)
HFM1		Primary ovarian failure
FSHR	FSH receptor	Hypergonadotrophic hypogonadism and ovarian hyperstimulation syndrome
FSHB	Follitropin subunit beta	Deficiency of FSH, primary amenorrhoea and infertility

Gene	Encoded Protein	Effect of Deficiency
FOXL2	Forkhead box L2	Isolated premature ovarian failure (POF3) associated with BPES type I; FOXL2
FMR1	Fragile X mental retardation	402C --> G mutations associated with human granulosa cell tumours
GNRH1	Gonadotropin releasing hormone	Premature ovarian failure (POF1) associated with premutations
GNRHR	GnRH receptor	Normosmic hypogonadotrophic hypogonadism
KAL1	Kallmann syndrome	Hypogonadotrophic hypogonadism
KISS1R ; GPR54	KISS1 receptor	Hypogonadotrophic hypogonadism and insomnia, X-linked Kallmann syndrome (KAL1)
LHB	Luteinizing hormone beta polypeptide	Hypogonadotrophic hypogonadism
LHCGR	LH/choriogonadotrophin receptor	Hypogonadism and pseudohermaphroditism
DAX1	Dosage-sensitive sex reversal, adrenal hypoplasia critical region, on chromosome X, gene 1	Hypergonadotrophic hypogonadism (luteinizing hormone resistance)
NR5A1; SF1	Steroidogenic factor 1	X-linked congenital adrenal hypoplasia with hypogonadotrophic hypogonadism; dosage-sensitive male-to-female sex reversal
POF1B	Premature ovarian failure 1B	46,XY male-to-female sex reversal and streak gonads and congenital lipoid adrenal hyperplasia; 46,XX gonadal dysgenesis and 46,XX primary ovarian insufficiency
PROK2	Prokineticin	Hypergonadotrophic, primary amenorrhea (POF2B)
PROKR2	Prokineticin receptor 2	Normosmic hypogonadotrophic hypogonadism and Kallmann syndrome (KAL4)
RSPO1	R-spondin family, member 1	Kallmann syndrome (KAL3)
SRY	Sex-determining region Y	46,XX, female-to-male sex reversal (individuals contain testes)
SOX9	SRY-related HMB-box gene 9	Mutations lead to 46,XY females; translocations lead to 46,XX males
STAG3	Stromal antigen 3	Autosomal 46,XY male-to-female sex reversal (campomelic dysplasia)
TAC3	Tachykinin 3	Premature ovarian failure
TACR3	Tachykinin receptor 3	Normosmic hypogonadotrophic hypogonadism
ZP1	Zona pellucida glycoprotein 1	Normosmic hypogonadotrophic hypogonadism

Investigations

Assessment of Ovulation

Ovulation is usually inferred when a woman reports regular cycles.

If there is doubt, progesterone level greater than 3 ng/mL is indicative of ovulation.

In the absence of pregnancy, progesterone production decreases after that.

Sonographic confirmation of follicle rupture with serial ultrasonography can also be performed.

Correlation with serum estradiol, LH, and progesterone levels are helpful.

Basal body temperature charts can be used to predict ovulation.

A basal body thermometer measures the slight rise in temperature that occurs immediately after ovulation.

However, most patients and physicians prefer to use urinary ovulation predictor kits as they are more accurate and easier to administer.

The LH surge in the serum will last for 36 hours and ovulation occurs 12 hours after the peak of the surge.

Therefore ovulation will occur within 24 hours of detecting the LH surge in urine.

False positives can occur in women who are perimenopausal and in women who have polycystic ovary syndrome (PCOS), as serum LH levels can be elevated in both of these situations.

Polycystic Ovarian Syndrome (PCOS)

Diagnostic criteria for PCOS have been defined in the Rotterdam Criteria published in 2003.

To make the diagnosis of PCOS, two out of the following three criteria are necessary:

– Oligoovulation or anovulation.

– Clinical and/or biochemical evidence of hyperandrogenism, such as hirsutism, acne, male-pattern baldness on exam or laboratory evaluation demonstrating elevated total testosterone, or free testosterone.

– Polycystic ovaries demonstrated on ultrasound.

Physical examination typically reveals excess male-pattern hair growth, predominantly in the midline.

Acne may be the only sign of hyperandrogenism in teenagers and Asian women.

Acanthosis nigricans is a raised, velvety hyperpigmentation of the skin seen on the dorsal surface of the neck and intertriginous areas, and is a marker of insulin resistance.

Obesity is seen in 50-75% of women with PCOS; however, many women with PCOS are thin.

Health consequences seen in women with PCOS include obesity, diabetes, dyslipidemia, hypertension, heart disease, endometrial hyperplasia, and infertility.

Laboratory assessment includes TSH, prolactin, FSH and estradiol, and 17-hydroxyprogesterone levels.

A total testosterone level is helpful to distinguish a tumor, but it is often normal or only slightly elevated in PCOS.

Free testosterone assay is imprecise, and is therefore often not recommended.

DHEAS is produced primarily by the adrenal gland and testing is not recommended unless there is concern about an adrenal tumor.

DHEAS is elevated in only 25% of women with PCOS.

LH/FSH ratio is only elevated (more than 2-fold) in 50-60% of women with PCOS and is non-diagnostic, and therefore it is not recommended.

Ultrasound criteria to diagnose PCOS include the presence of more than 12 follicles of 2 to 9 mm in diameter and increased ovarian volume of $>10 \text{ mL}^3$.

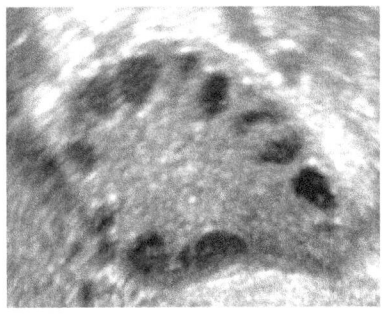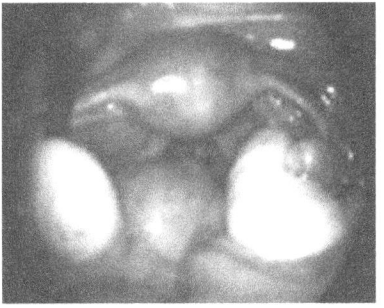

Ultrasonography   **Laparoscopy**

Polycystic Ovarian Syndrome (PCOS)

Ovarian Reserve

The level of ovarian reserve and the age of the female partner are the most important prognostic factors in the fertility workup.

Ovarian reserve is most commonly evaluated by checking a cycle day 3 FSH and estradiol level.

Normal ovarian function is indicated when the FSH level is less than 10 mIU/mL and the estradiol level is less than 65 pg/mL.

In cases where the patient is 35 years or older, dynamic ovarian reserve testing may be indicated.

The most common test used is the clomiphene citrate challenge test (CCCT).

A serum FSH and estradiol level is drawn on cycle day 3.

Clomiphene citrate (CC) 100 mg by mouth is administered on cycle days 5-9 and a serum FSH level is drawn again on day 10.

An FSH level greater than 10 is associated with decreased fertility and lower pregnancy rates.

Other tests of ovarian reserve include antral follicle counts, ovarian volume, inhibin B, and antimüllerian hormone.

However, most of these have not been found to be of adequate sensitivity, specificity, or positive predictive value when applying cutoffs across all age groups for pregnancy.

They are predictive of response to ovulation induction medications.

Treatment

Induction of Ovulation

Ovulation induction is the appropriate treatment for infertile patients who have dysfunction of the hypothalamic-pituitary-ovarian axis.

Clomiphene Citrate (CC)

The chemical formula for CC is 2-[p - (2-chloro-1,2-difhenylvinyl) phenoxy] triethylamine dihydrogen citrate.

CC is a nonsteroidal selective estrogen receptor modulator (SERM) capable of interacting with estrogen receptor binding proteins in a manner similar to estrogen but in a more prolonged way.

Therefore, CC behaves similar to an antiestrogen.

CC has been in clinical use since the early 1960s.

Its mechanism of action is still not well understood, but it competes for the estrogen receptor at the hypothalamus, pituitary, and ovarian levels.

Because of the action at the estrogen-receptor level within the hypothalamus, CC alleviates the negative feedback effect exerted by endogenous estrogens.

As a result, CC normalizes the GnRH release; therefore, the secretion of FSH and LH is capable of normalized follicular recruitment, selection, and development to reestablish the normal process of ovulation.

The standard dose of CC is 50 mg PO qd for 5 days, starting on the menstrual cycle day 3-5 or after progestin-induced bleeding.

As an antiestrogen, CC requires that the patient have some circulating estrogen levels; otherwise, the patient will not respond to the treatment.

The CC response is monitored using pelvic ultrasonography starting on menstrual cycle day 12.

The follicle should develop to a diameter of 23-24 mm before a spontaneous LH surge occurs.

BBT can be used to observe the thermogenic shift induced by the early secretion of progesterone.

The only disadvantage with BBT is that in many instances, the shift does not occur in a clear way, and the patient misses the time of ovulation.

While BBT is an inexpensive way to monitor ovulation, it is often impractical.

Urinary monitoring of the LH surge (eg, with an LH Predictor Kit) can be a substitute for BBT.

The patient should start monitoring the urinary LH secretion daily starting on menstrual cycle day 12.

Ovulation usually occurs within the 32-40 hours after the indicative color change.

Serum LH determination is more precise, especially when performed in combination with pelvic ultrasonography.

Because of the antiestrogenic effect, CC may thicken the cervical mucus, creating an iatrogenic cervical factor that can be responsible for the lack of pregnancy in a patient who has otherwise ovulated.

Other adverse effects associated with CC are hot flashes, scotomas, dryness of the vagina, headache, and ovarian hyperstimulation, which, although rare, has been reported in patients who are sensitive to CC.

The principal indications for CC use are oligomenorrhea, especially PCOS, and for patients with slight menstrual irregularities.

The use of CC is contraindicated in cases of ovarian cyst, pregnancy, and liver disease.

Its use is controversial in patients with a history of breast cancer.

Tamoxifen

Tamoxifen is another SERM, similar to clomiphene that is typically used in the treatment of breast cancer.

Tamoxifen can also be used for ovulation induction.

But, unlike clomiphene, it does not have an anti-estrogenic effect on the uterus.

However, some studies indicate there may be an increased risk for miscarriage with tamoxifen use.

The typical dose is 20 mg daily for 5 days in the early follicular phase, similar to clomiphene.

Success rates with its use are similar to those of clomiphene.

Aromatase Inhibitors

Aromatase inhibitors inhibit the action of the enzyme aromatase, which converts androgens into estrogens by a process called aromatization.

As a result, estrogen levels are dramatically reduced, releasing the hypothalamic-pituitary axis from its negative feedback.

Aromatase inhibitors are FDA approved for treatment of postmenopausal breast cancer, but not for ovulation induction.

When used in the early follicular phase, letrozole inhibits estrogen synthesis, thereby causing enhanced GnRH pulsatility and consequent FSH and inhibin stimulation.

This results in normal or enhanced follicular recruitment without the risk of multiple ovulation and ovarian hyperstimulation syndrome.

Letrozole has a very short half-life (45 hours) and, therefore, is quickly cleared from the body.

For this reason, it is less likely to adversely affect the endometrium and cervical mucus.

In a recent meta-analysis, letrozole was found to be as effective as other methods of ovulation induction.

The usual dose for letrozole ovulation induction is 2.5 mg on cycle days 3-7, however, the optimal dosage and length of administration is under investigation.

Aromatase inhibitors are generally well tolerated.

The main side effects are hot flushes, gastrointestinal events (nausea and vomiting), headache, back pain, and leg cramps.

These adverse effects were reported in older women with advanced breast cancer who were given the drugs on a daily basis over several months.

In younger women taking them at lower doses for a short period of time, fewer adverse effects are noted.

The use of aromatase inhibitors for ovulation induction in premenopausal women is controversial due to the possibility of fetal toxicity and fetal malformations.

Furthermore, based on the half-life, administration in the early follicular phase should result in clearance of the aromatase inhibitors before implantation takes place.

<u>Dopamine Agonists</u>

Dopamine agonists are agents that can be used for restoration of ovulation in women with galactorrhea or hyperprolactinemia.

Two agents are available for use, bromocriptine and cabergoline.

Cabergoline is more selective, as it binds specifically to dopamine 2 receptors on the lactotrope cells, and thus has fewer side effects.

Dopamine agonists function like dopamine; they suppress prolactin synthesis and release from the pituitary.

By normalizing the prolactin level, the hypothalamic-pituitary-ovarian axis can return to normal function.

The two drugs are administered slightly differently, although a key component of the use of both is to start at a low dose and titrate up slowly.

Bromocriptine is given at an initial dose of 1.25 mg at bedtime for one week, then increased to twice daily for a month.

A prolactin level can be checked at that time, and if not within normal range, the dose can be increased to 2.5 mg, and then 5 mg if needed.

Cabergoline is given at a dose of 0.25 mg twice a week.

This is increased to 0.5 mg, and then 1.0 mg, twice a week, if after a month at each dose the prolactin level is not yet in normal range.

A response to treatment can be seen by a drop in the serum prolactin level 2-3 weeks after the initiation of therapy.

Normalization of serum prolactin levels should be accompanied by normal menstrual cycles.

Dopamine agonists are successful for treating anovulation; 80% of women will ovulate after correction of hyperprolactinemia, with cumulative pregnancy rates of 70-80%.

Adverse effects for both drugs include dizziness, nausea, and hypotension.

Cabergoline is better tolerated, as it is the more selective of the two drugs.

Both can be administered vaginally to improve tolerability.

Gonadotropins

Human menopausal gonadotropin (hMG) contains 75 U of FSH and 75 U of LH per mL, although the concentration may vary among batches.

In the 1980s, a pure form of FSH became available; urofollitropin contains 75 U of FSH.

The new generations of available gonadotropins are produced by genetically engineered mammalian cells (ie, Chinese hamster ovary cells), in which the gene coding for the alpha and beta FSH subunits has been inserted.

Recombinant LH may be added to recombinant FSH protocols as an alternative, particularly useful in patients with hypothalamic amenorrhea.

The administration of hMG and its derivatives should be under the direct supervision of a reproductive endocrinologist.

An ultrasonography unit and an endocrine laboratory capable of performing daily determinations of E_2, FSH, and LH are necessary.

Multiple adverse effects and complications may occur during the use of the gonadotropins, including

–Multiple pregnancy (24-33%).

–Ectopic pregnancy (5-8%).

–Miscarriages (15-21%).

–Ovarian torsion and rupture.

–Ovarian hyperstimulation syndrome (OHSS).

The increase of ovarian cancer associated with infertility might be due to the use of fertility drugs.

OHSS is an iatrogenic condition that occurs in patients undergoing ovulation induction with hMG or controlled ovarian hyperstimulation for assisted reproductive technologies.

The pathophysiology is not well understood, but a massive extravascular accumulation of fluid occurs that is associated with depletion of intravascular volume responsible for dehydration, hemoconcentration, and electrolyte imbalance (hyponatremia, hyperkalemia).

OHSS can be mild, moderate, or severe.

Mild OHSS is characterized by ovarian enlargement (up to 5-12 cm in diameter), minimal ascites, and weight gain of less than 10 lb.

Moderate OHSS is characterized by ovarian enlargement (5-12 cm in diameter) moderate ascites, nausea, vomiting, abdominal discomfort, and weight gain greater than 10 lb.

Severe OHSS is characterized by easily palpable ovaries, severe ascites, nausea, vomiting, diarrhea, shortness of breath, hydrothorax, peripheral edema, oliguria, hemoconcentration (eg, hematocrit level >48% and hemoglobin level >16 g), and creatinine level greater than 1.6 mg/dL.

Renal failure and thrombosis can occur if the patient is not treated correctly.

Some patients have a greater risk of developing OHSS.

They are usually young patients with a history of PCOS or oligo-ovulation who responded with elevated E_2 levels (3000 pc/mL) and multiple follicles (>15) and patients in whom the ovulation has been triggered by the administration of exogenous hCG.

OHSS usually has 2 phases; the first phase develops between the second and seventh day after ovulation, and the second phase only occurs if the patient becomes pregnant.

OHSS is self-limited, and the symptoms subside within 2-6 weeks.

Patients with mild and moderate OHSS are treated at home with bedrest and strict control of fluid intake and output.

If a weight gain greater than 2 lb occurs, the patient should be evaluated to determine if hospitalization is required.

Patients with severe OHSS are often hospitalized and confined to bed, with strict control of fluid intake and output.

Intravenous fluids (ie, isotonic sodium chloride solution) must be administered until hemodilution is achieved.

If the urinary output remains low, albumin 25% (50 mL/h IV for 4 h) has been effective in promoting diuresis.

Transvaginal or abdominal paracentesis should be performed if the patient becomes uncomfortable.

Because of the risk of thrombosis, heparin (5000 U SC q12h) is recommended.

Some have had success treating severe OHSS on an outpatient basis by performing aggressive transvaginal paracentesis with good outcomes.

hMG and its derivatives are indicated for ovulation induction in patients with primary amenorrhea due to hypopituitarism and in patients with secondary amenorrhea who did not respond to CC ovulation induction.

For the past 20 years, hMG and its derivatives have been the first choice for controlled ovarian hyperstimulation in assisted reproductive technologies.

Human Chorionic Gonadotropins (hCG)

hCG is available in two preparations, similar to the gonadotropins: purified urinary hCG and recombinant hCG.

hCG is used for triggering final follicular maturation and/or ovulation.

It can provide this function because it is very similar in structure to LH.

Both hormones contain the same alpha subunit; however, the beta subunit is also very similar, so hCG can bind to and activate the LH receptor.

When used to trigger ovulation, a dose of 5,000-10,000 IU of urinary hCG is typically given by intramuscular or subcutaneous injection; other doses have also been used.

The dose of recombinant hCG that is used is 250 mcg, given by subcutaneous injection, which is roughly equivalent to 6,000 IU of hCG activity.

There is no difference in pregnancy outcomes between urinary and recombinant forms.

Lower doses have been suggested as a means for reducing the risk of OHSS.

However, the efficacy of this approach has not been proven in randomized controlled trials.

When hCG is used as an ovulation trigger, ultrasound is used to monitor follicle size and time administration of hCG.

Ovulation will occur 36-44 hours following the injection.

Gonadotropin Releasing Hormone (GnRH)

Synthetic GnRH has a chemical composition similar to native GnRH and is indicated for patients with hypothalamic dysfunction, especially those who do not respond to CC.

This drug is administered in a pulsatile fashion every 60-120 minutes, intravenously or subcutaneously using a delivery pump.

The starting dose is 5 mcg per pulse intravenously or 5-25 mcg subcutaneously.

The administration on GnRH should be extended throughout the luteal phase, or this should be supplemented with the administration of exogenous hCG.

Monitoring folliculogenesis is simpler than using hMG.

Pelvic ultrasonography can be used once a week until the dominant follicle is detected; once this occurs, ultrasonography can be used more frequently until ovulation occurs.

Determination of serum E_2 and LH levels can also be performed.

Gonadotropin Releasing Hormone (GnRH) Antagonists

Similar to the GnRH agonists, GnRH antagonists were developed by modification of the native GnRH protein.

Two products are marketed for use in the US: cetrorelix and ganirelix.

Both function to antagonize GnRH by binding and blocking the GnRH receptor from signaling.

They are used in controlled ovarian stimulation IVF cycles to prevent a premature LH surge.

Both compounds are formulated as a 0.25 mg subcutaneous injection that is given daily to suppress the LH surge.

Treatment is typically started when the lead follicle reaches a diameter of 14 mm, or when estradiol levels reach 400 pg/mL.

The antagonist is then continued daily until ovulation trigger.

Cetrorelix can also be given as a single dose of 3 mg subcutaneously on day 8 or 9 of stimulation; this may need to be repeated if stimulation continues for more than 3 additional days.

Routine monitoring of controlled ovarian stimulation with serial estradiol levels and ultrasounds is performed; one can anticipate a blunting of the estradiol response as a result of starting antagonist therapy.

Treatment of Polycystic Ovarian Syndrome (PCOS)

There are multiple treatments available for women with PCOS desiring to conceive.

Weight loss for obese women is important, not only for improving chances of ovulation, but also for reducing the risks during pregnancy.

CC is the first-line drug for treatment of anovulation with 22% conception rates per cycle, which is comparable to normal cycle fecundity.

Side effects include hot flushes, moodiness, a 10% rate of twin gestation, and 0.5% rate of triplet gestation.

Metformin is an insulin-sensitizing agent that has been used with off-label indication in the treatment of PCOS.

However, the use of metformin as an adjunct to other therapies in subsets of infertile women with PCOS has yet to be determined.

Gonadotropin therapy for ovulation induction in women with PCOS has been shown to be successful with pregnancy rates of approximately 22%.

OHSS remains a significant concern due multiple follicular development and hypersensitive ovaries.

Ovarian drilling involves drilling 3 to 10 holes per ovary at laparoscopy using electrocautery or laser.

In women with PCOS who are resistant to CC, ovarian drilling results in ovulation rates of 75 to 85%, which are similar to results seen with adding metformin for CC-resistant women.

Risks of the surgery include ovarian adhesions and ovarian failure if too many holes are drilled.

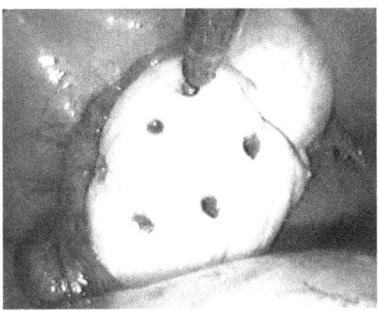

Laparoscopic Ovarian Drilling

Treatment of Prolactinomas

The goal of treatment for women with a prolactinoma is to normalize prolactin and therefore restore gonadotropin levels to normal in order to facilitate menstrual cyclicity.

Medical therapy involves the use of dopamine agonists to suppress prolactin secretion.

The most commonly used dopamine agonist is bromocriptine.

Cabergoline is a newer option and has fewer side effects.

The two drugs are administered slightly differently, although a key component of the use of both is to start at a low dose and titrate up slowly.

A response to treatment can be seen by a drop in the serum prolactin level 2-3 weeks after the initiation of therapy.

Once the prolactin level is normalized, ovulation will be restored within a few months.

Macroadenomas can be treated medically, but surgery is often the preferred method for large masses.

FALLOPIAN TUBES

The fallopian tubes (also referred to as uterine tubes or oviducts) are uterine appendages located bilaterally at the superior portion of the cavity.

The fallopian tubes exit the uterus through an area known as the cornua and form a connection between the endometrial and peritoneal cavities.

Each tube is approximately 10 cm in length and 1 cm in diameter and is situated within a portion of the broad ligament called the mesosalpinx.

The distal portion of the fallopian tube ends in an orientation encircling the ovary.

The fallopian tube has 4 parts.

– The first segment, closest to the uterus, is called the isthmus.

– The second segment is the ampulla, which becomes more dilated in diameter and is the typical place of fertilization.

– The final segment, furthest from the uterus, is the infundibulum.

– The infundibulum gives rise to the fimbriae, fingerlike projections that are responsible for catching the egg that is released by the ovary.

The arterial supply to the fallopian tubes is from branches of the uterine and ovarian arteries, located within the mesosalpinx.

Lymphatic drainage of the fallopian tubes is through the iliac and aortic nodes.

The nerve supply to the fallopian tubes is via both sympathetic and parasympathetic fibers; sensory fibers run from thoracic segments 11-12 and lumbar segment 1.

Microscopic Anatomy

The tubal mucosa has many folds, or plicae, which are most evident in the ampulla; a smooth muscular layer surrounds the mucosa.

Within the mucosa of the uterine tubes, 3 different cell types exist:

– Columnar ciliated epithelial cells (25%).

– Secretory cells (60%).

– Narrow peg cells (< 10%).

Functional Anatomy

The released (ovulated) oocyte is guided by waving movements of the infundibulum and fimbriae; muscular peristalsis moves the egg through the fallopian tube.

Fertilization usually occurs in the distal third of the fallopian tube adjacent to ovary (ampulla).

Peristalsis moves the fertilized oocyte through the tubal isthmus and into the uterus for implantation.

Estradiol promotes growth, proliferation and ciliogenesis.

Both estradiol and progesterone increase contractions of the muscular layer to promote transport of the oocyte and fertilized zygote.

The composition of the oviductal fluid is crucial to the survival and development of the zygote; it is tightly regulated by the secretory epithelial cells.

The fluid is enriched in sodium and potassium; oviductal fluid also is enriched in lactic acid and bicarbonate, which are important for cleavage of fertilized eggs or zygotes.

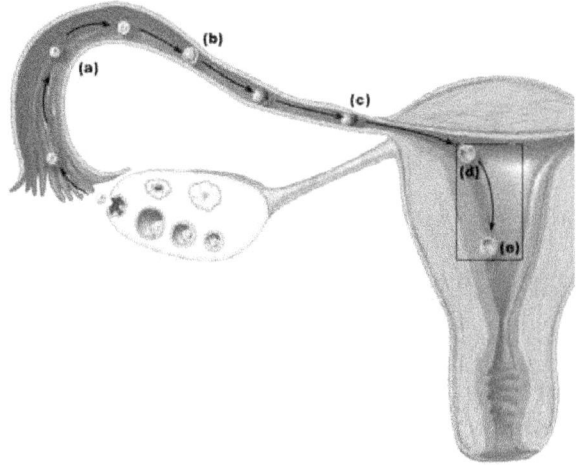

Fallopian (Uterine) Tubes

FERTILIZATION

The fallopian tubes, or oviducts, function as conduits for the oocyte and spermatozoa, and they provide nutrients for the gametes and early embryo, as well as serving as the site of fertilization.

Ciliated cells at the open, fimbriated end (ostium) direct the oocyte into the infundibulum and down through the ampulla.

Fertilization usually occurs in the distal third of the fallopian tube adjacent to ovary (ampulla).

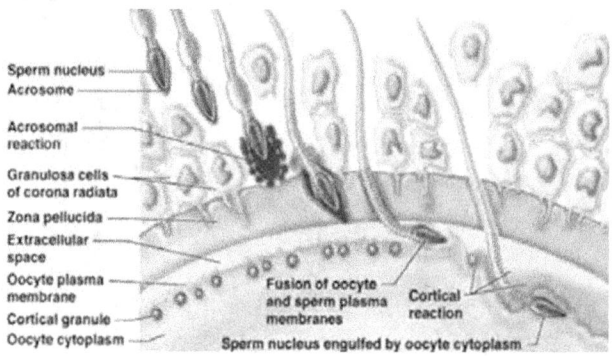

Fertilization

The zygote is kept in the fallopian tube for about three days by the spastic contractions of the estrogen-dominated isthmus; as progesterone increases, muscle tone decreases.

Once the zygote divides it is called an embryo; while still in the fallopian tube, the embryo undergoes cleavage division (1-cell to 8-cell), compaction and blastocyst formation before it reaches the uterus.

The inner cell mass of the embryo becomes the fetus and the outer cells become the placenta and fetal membranes.

Peristalsis moves the fertilized oocyte through the tubal isthmus and into the uterus for implantation.

Approximately seven days after fertilization, the blastocyst bursts from the zona pellucida (hatching) and implants in the wall of the uterus.

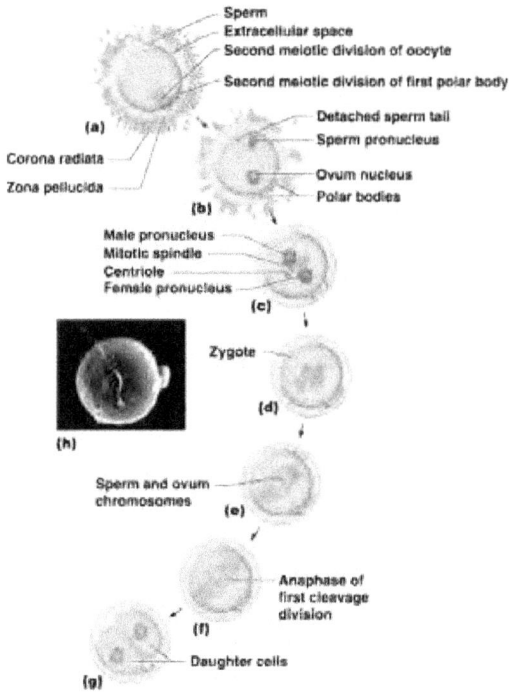

Embryo Cleavage

TUBAL FACTORS OF INFERTILITY

The fallopian tubes play an important role in reproduction.

After ovulation, the fimbriae pick up the oocyte from the peritoneal fluid that has accumulated in the cul-de-sac.

The epithelial cilia transport the oocyte up to the ampulla.

The capacitated spermatozoa are transported from the endometrium through the cornual section and advanced through the fallopian tube down into the ampulla, where fertilization occurs.

The embryo initiates its early cleaving stages and is propelled upward to arrive at the endometrial cavity at the blastocyst stage.

Causes

Abnormalities or damage to the fallopian tube interferes with fertility and is responsible for abnormal implantation (eg, ectopic pregnancy).

Obstruction of the distal end of the fallopian tubes results in accumulation of the normally secreted tubal fluid, creating distention of the tube with subsequent damage of the epithelial cilia (hydrosalpinx).

Other tubal factors associated with infertility are either congenital or acquired.

Congenital absence of the fallopian tubes can be due to spontaneous torsion in utero followed by necrosis and reabsorption.

Elective tubal ligation and salpingectomy are acquired causes.

The uterus, ovaries, and fallopian tubes share the same space within the peritoneal cavity.

Anatomical defects or physiologic dysfunctions of the peritoneal cavity, including infection, adhesions, and adnexal masses, may cause infertility.

PID, peritoneal adhesions secondary to previous pelvic surgery, endometriosis, and ovarian cyst rupture all compromise the motility of the fallopian tubes or produce blockage of the fimbriae with development of hydrosalpinx.

Large myomas, pelvic masses, or blockage of the cul-de-sac interferes with the accumulation of peritoneal fluid and interferes with the normal oocyte pickup mechanism.

Peri-ovarian adhesions interfere with the normal oocyte release at ovulation, becoming a mechanical factor for infertility.

Pelvic Inflammatory Disease (PID)

PID has been associated with gonorrhea infection for more than a century.

While gonorrhea still plays an important role in tubal disease, it has been surpassed by chlamydia.

Westrom reported a 21% incidence of infertility in a group of Swedish women who were diagnosed with PID.

The rate of damage to the fallopian tubes increases with subsequent PID episodes, from 34% for the first episode to 54% in women with second and third episodes.

PID can be diagnosed clinically and confirmed by results from cervical culture and serologic antibody assays for gonorrhea and chlamydia.

In many instances, a patient never recalls having had an acute PID episode; however, years later, the incidental finding of tubal obstruction after HSG or laparoscopy may be the only indication of previous disease.

Endometriosis

Endometriosis remains an enigmatic disease that affects women during their reproductive years.

The incidence increases with patient age and low parity.

Pelvic pain and reproductive failure are the 2 major complaints of patients with endometriosis.

Although a gene defect has not yet been identified for endometriosis, a genetic link seems probable based on the observation of chromosomal defects in endometriotic tissue and the observation of a 7-fold increased risk of endometriosis in patients with a family history of the disease.

Endometriotic lesions vary from microscopic to macroscopic.

Classic endometriosis appears as bluish-black pigments, (ie, "powder-burn lesions") that affect the peritoneal surfaces of the bladder, ovary, fallopian tubes, cul-de-sac, and bowel.

Nonclassic endometriosis may appear as red, tan, or white lesions and vesicles.

The final diagnosis should be confirmed by demonstrating endometrial stroma and glands in biopsy tissue.

The incidence of endometriosis in primary and secondary infertility varies according to the population studied with an incidence rate of 26% and 13%, respectively.

Severe endometriosis with damage to the fallopian tubes and ovaries due to adhesions or the presence of endometriomas is an obvious cause of infertility.

The hypothesis that minimal and mild endometriosis may cause infertility is controversial.

Minimal and mild endometriosis is hypothesized to reduce fertility by the following mechanisms:

- Increased peritoneal macrophages increases phagocytosis of the sperm.

- Decreased sperm binding to the zona pellucida.

- Proliferation of peritoneal lymphocytes.

- Increased cytokinin levels.

- Increased immunoglobulin production.

- Embryo toxic serum.

- Defective natural killer activity.

- Endometriosis has been associated with ovulatory disorders such as LPD, oligo-ovulation, and LUF syndrome.

Although pelvic pain appears to be a common symptom of endometriosis, in some patients, endometriosis is an incidental finding discovered during diagnostic laparoscopy for evaluation of infertility.

Investigations

The 2 most frequent tests used for diagnosis of tubal pathology are hysterosalpingogram and laparoscopy.

Hysterosalpingogram (HSG)

HSG is the most frequently used diagnostic tool to evaluate the endometrial cavity and fallopian tubes.

Some have tried to displace the role of HSG in the evaluation of infertility; however, a meticulous and well-executed procedure, performed under fluoroscopy, provides accurate information about:

– Endocervical canal.

– Diameter and configuration of the internal os.

– Endometrial cavity.

– Uterine/tubal junction (cornual ostium).

– Diameter, location, and direction of the fallopian tubes.

– Status of the fimbriae.

– Spill into the endometrial cavity.

Furthermore, the HSG provides indirect evidence of pelvic adhesions and uterine, ovarian, or adnexal masses.

The HSG should be performed during the early follicular phase; at this time, the endometrium is thin and the HSG provides better delineation of minor defects.

In addition, the possibility of accidental irradiation to the fetus in an undiagnosed pregnancy is eliminated.

The cervix is cleansed with a povidone-iodine solution to avoid the transfer of bacteria to the endometrial cavity during the procedure.

A breakaway vaginal speculum is used so it can be removed before injection of the radiopaque medium.

A single-tooth tenaculum is used to apply traction of the uterus and to correct any anteroflexion or retroflexion that yields suboptimal images.

A Jarcho-type metal cannula with a plastic adjustable acorn or a balloon HSG catheter is used for the injection of radiocontrast media.

The use of water-based contrast media is preferable to oil-based media to avoid the risks of oil embolism and granuloma formation.

Consider a short course of prophylactic antibiotic use if there is a suspicion of previous tubal infection.

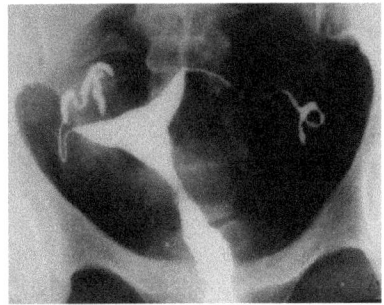
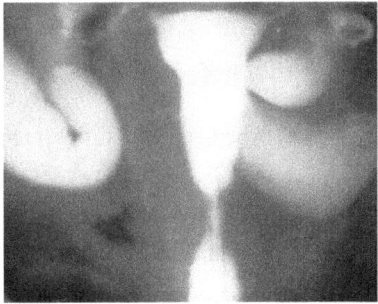

Normal   **Hydrosalpinx**

Hysterosalpingogram (HSG)

Laparoscopy

The laparoscope is one of the greatest developments in gynecologic instrumentation.

Its origin dates to the pioneering work of Jacobaeus in 1910.

The laparoscope was first used to visualize the pelvic cavity.

The procedure was abandoned in the 1930s because of fatal complications.

In the 1950s, a new generation of laparoscope was developed using a fiberoptic technique; later, safer electrocautery techniques resurrected the application and use of operative laparoscopy, especially for sterilization purposes and for diagnosis of ectopic pregnancy.

In 1970, Semm advanced the field of operative laparoscopy with the development of numerous accessory instruments.

Semm opened the doors to new surgical applications and forever changed the traditional way of practicing gynecologic surgery.

Laparoscopy is not part of the routine infertility evaluation.

It is used when abnormalities are found on ultrasonography, HSG, or suspected by symptomology.

A direct view into the abdominal cavity allows for inspecting the ovaries, fallopian tubes, and uterus.

Laparoscopy sometimes uncovers adhesions which can interfere with the fallopian tube's ability to pick up the oocyte from the ovary.

Tubal patency can be assessed along with the laparoscopy.

Typically, 2 to 4 small incisions are made on the skin to insert the laparoscope and other instruments as required.

Because of the added risks of surgery, need for anesthesia, and operative cost, it is only used when clearly indicated.

Laparoscopy is contraindicated in patients with probable bowel obstruction (ileus) and bowel distention, cardiopulmonary disease, or shock due to internal bleeding.

Because of the risk of bowel perforation, uterine and pelvic vessel injury, and bladder trauma, an experienced surgeon must perform the procedure.

Relative contraindications include massive obesity, large abdominal mass or advanced pregnancy, severe pelvic adhesions, and peritonitis.

The 1996 American Society for Reproductive Medicine's Revised Classification of Endometriosis is a staging system to standardize the degree of endometriosis and facilitate communication about the amount of disease.

Unfortunately, the staging system does not correlate with a women's chance of conception following therapy.

ASRM's classification of endometriosis bases the determination of the stage or degree of endometrial involvement on a weighted point system at the time of laparoscopy.

The number, size and location of endometrial implants, endometriomas and/or adhesions are noted.

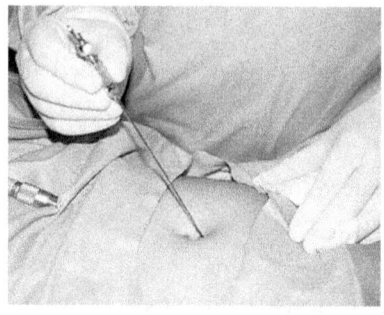

Veress Needle Insertion

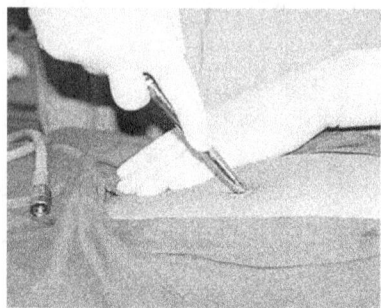

Primary Trocar Insertion

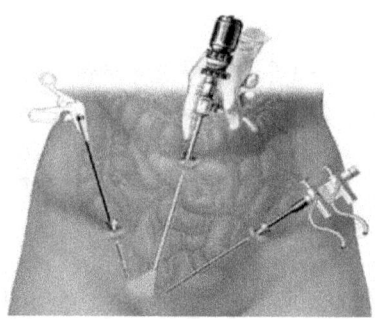

Accessory Trocars Insertion

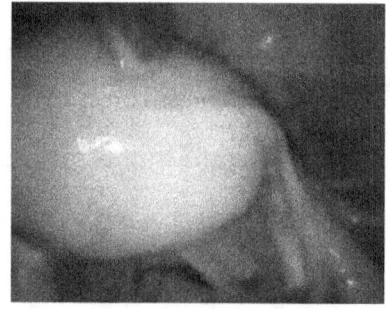

Pelvic Exploration

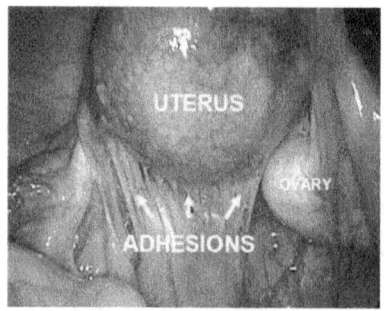

Pelvic Adhesions

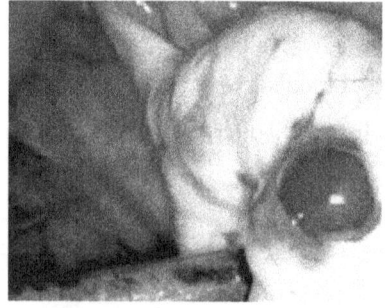

Ovarian Endometriosis

Laparoscopy

Treatment

The treatment of tubal-factor infertility underwent major changes, especially when microsurgery became available.

Tubal reconstruction was the only hope for those patients before assisted reproductive therapy became available.

Because of the intimate relationship between the fallopian tubes and the other pelvic organs and because, in the great majority of the cases, peritoneal pathology involves tubal pathology, the treatments of these factors are discussed together.

Tubal and peritoneal factor infertility treatment requires a good surgeon who is skilled in currently available techniques.

The patient's age and the severity of the tubal pathology play important roles in the selection of patients, as do any other infertility issues such as the presence of endometriosis and severe pelvic adhesions.

Before surgery, the HSG films and results of previous laparoscopies should be thoroughly reviewed to decide on the type of surgical technique that is required and to explain to the patient the expected degree of success and risks involved with the procedure.

Tubal obstruction and lysis of adhesions can be corrected through laparotomy, operative laparoscopy, and, in special circumstances, through operative hysteroscopy and tubal cannulation.

Laparotomy is indicated with severe pelvic adhesions that compromise the bowel, ovaries, and tubes, with obliteration of the cul-de-sac.

The aim of the procedure is to correct what is necessary to allow the normal transport of the gametes; complete restoration of the anatomy is not intended.

Lysis of adhesions should be meticulous, using hydrodissection and fine instruments.

Blunt dissection should be avoided.

Constant irrigation with Ringer lactate solution and heparin prevents fibrin formation.

Meticulous hemostasis is imperative.

Operative hysteroscopy associated with tubal cannulation is helpful to treat cornual obstruction.

Fimbrial phimosis and periadnexal disease can be treated with laparoscopy.

The pregnancy rate after salpingolysis is 50-60% during the first year after treatment.

Fimbrioplasty for fimbria agglutination or phimosis without destruction of the cilial epithelium is equally successful.

The incidence of ectopic pregnancy after surgery is in the range of 5%.

Treatment of hydrosalpinx (distal tubal obstruction) with salpingostomy can be performed through microsurgery or operative laparoscopy.

No difference in the pregnancy rate occurs if a skillful microsurgeon or laparoscopist performs the salpingostomy.

The success of the procedure is related to the diameter of the hydrosalpinx and to the damage to the cilial epithelium.

If the cilial epithelium has been destroyed, the outcome of the procedure is poor, and it is better to perform a salpingectomy in preparation for future IVF.

The pregnancy rate fluctuates from 20-35%, and the expected ectopic pregnancy rate is as high as 20%.

Before treating cornual obstruction, the diagnosis should be confirmed; in many cases, cornual obstruction diagnosed on HSG represents simple cornual spasm.

Before performing a tubocornual anastomosis, the patient should have a laparoscopy associated with tubal cannulation by hysteroscopy.

If one tube remains open, anastomosis is not needed because pregnancy can be achieved in 50% of cases.

The success rate of tubocornual anastomosis ranges from 20-58%, the ectopic pregnancy rate is 5-7%.

If the obstruction is caused by salpingitis isthmica nodosa or fibrosis, the best results are achieved through IVF.

The surgeon should consider that the patient is better served with a single well-functioning fallopian tube than with 2 defective tubes, which elicits an increased risk for ectopic pregnancy or recurrence of pelvic adhesions.

If the fallopian tubes are beyond repair, bilateral salpingectomy with destruction of the cornual area is recommended in preparation for IVF.

Treatment of Endometriosis

Endometriosis treatment may be divided according to the severity of the disease and patient needs.

Four alternatives are currently available to treat endometriosis: expectant therapy, surgical intervention, medical treatment, and combined therapy.

Expectant therapy should be based on a complete workup with diagnosis of very early stages of the disease (minimal) in patients without clinical symptoms, ie, an incidental finding.

A second-look laparoscopy is required for follow-up within 6-18 months.

Surgical treatment should be directed at destroying the disease using electrocoagulation, laser vaporization, endocoagulation, or excision.

Most surgical treatment for endometriosis is currently performed through operative laparoscopy.

Laparotomy has been relegated to the treatment of severe disease or if a need for hysterectomy arises.

Medical treatment is directed toward suppressing estrogen production by the ovary.

Depending on the therapeutic agent and the duration of treatment, endometriosis can be treated with oral contraceptives, progestins (eg, Medroxyprogesterone acetate), androgens (eg, danazol), or GnRH agonists (eg, Leuprolide acetate).

Combined medical and surgical treatments are usually used for the treatment of severe endometriosis.

No consensus exists as to whether the medical treatment should precede surgery or vice versa.

Those who prefer medical treatment first argue that the size of the endometriosis decreases; therefore, surgery will be easier and shorter.

Those who prefer surgery first argue that because the size of endometriosis decreases, the operation is less than ideal and is associated with an increased chance for early recurrence.

Regardless of the treatment approach, establish a 6- to 12-month interval during which a spontaneous pregnancy is expected to occur.

For patients wishing to conceive, the medical approach is not indicated, as it delays treatment for infertility.

Medical treatment for minimal to mild disease has not been shown to be of benefit.

However, for women with moderate to severe endometriosis, surgical treatment then assisted reproductive therapy can be offered.

Assisted Reproduction Techniques (ART)

In vitro fertilization (IVF) consists of retrieving a preovulatory oocyte from the ovary and fertilizing it with sperm in the laboratory, with subsequent embryo transfer within the endometrial cavity.

Absence of the fallopian tubes and severe pelvic adhesions were the absolute indications for IVF, but they have been broadened.

Patients with a history of endometriosis unsuccessfully treated medically or surgically can undergo IVF.

Patients with husbands who have severe oligospermia or a history of obstructive azoospermia are also candidates for IVF.

Finally, patients who have failed more conservative therapies or with an unknown etiology of infertility may undergo IVF.

IVF generally requires a minimum of 50,000-500,000 motile sperm.

Harvesting eggs initially involves down-regulating the woman's pituitary with a GnRH agonist and then performing ovarian hyperstimulation.

Follicular development is monitored by ultrasonographic examination and by checking serum levels of estrogen and progesterone.

When the follicles are appropriately enlarged, a transvaginal follicular aspiration is performed.

A mean of 12 eggs are typically retrieved per cycle, and they are immediately placed in an agar of fallopian-tube medium.

After an incubation period of 3-6 hours, the sperm are added to the medium using approximately 100,000 sperm per oocyte.

After 48 hours, the embryos have usually reached the 3- to 8-cell stage.

Two to 4 embryos are usually implanted in the uterus, while the remaining embryos are frozen for future use.

Pregnancy rates are 10-45%.

Risks include multiple pregnancies and hyperstimulation syndrome.

Intracytoplasmic sperm injection (ICSI) involves the direct injection of a sperm into an egg under microscopy.

It is indicated in patients who have failed more conservative therapies or those with severe semen abnormalities including patients with sperm extracted directly from the epididymis or testicle.

Oocytes are processed with hyaluronidase to remove the cumulus mass and corona radiata.

A micropipette is used to hold the egg while a second micropipette injects the sperm.

The oocyte is positioned with the polar body at the 6-o'clock or 12-o'clock position, and the sperm is injected at the 3-o'clock position to minimize the risk of chromosomal damage in the egg.

After incubation for 48 hours, the embryo is implanted in the woman.

A 59% fertilization rate and a 35% pregnancy rate with the use of ICSI was reported.

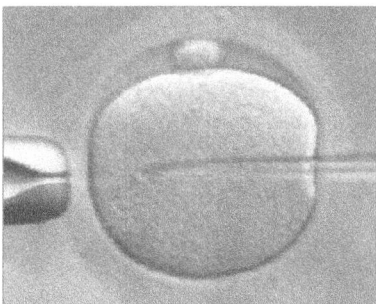

Intracytoplasmic Sperm Injection (ICSI)

UTERUS

The uterus is the inverted pear-shaped female reproductive organ that lies in the midline of the body, within the pelvis between the bladder and the rectum.

It is thick-walled and muscular, with a lining that, during reproductive years, changes in response to hormone stimulation throughout a woman's monthly cycle.

The uterus can be divided into 3 parts:

– The most inferior aspect is the cervix, and

– The bulk of the organ is called the body of the uterus (corpus uteri).

– Between these 2 is the isthmus, a short area of constriction.

The body of the uterus is globe-shaped and is typically situated in an anteverted position, at a 90° angle to the vagina.

The upper aspect of the body is dome-shaped and is called the fundus; it is typically the most muscular part of the uterus.

The body of the uterus is responsible for holding a pregnancy, and strong uterine wall contractions help to expel the fetus during labor and delivery.

The average weight of a nonpregnant, nulliparous uterus is approximately 40-50 g.

A multiparous uterus may weigh slightly more than this, with an upper limit of approximately 110 g.

A menopausal uterus is small and atrophied and typically weighs much less.

The uterine cavity is flattened and triangular; the uterine tubes enter the cavity bilaterally in the superolateral portion of the cavity.

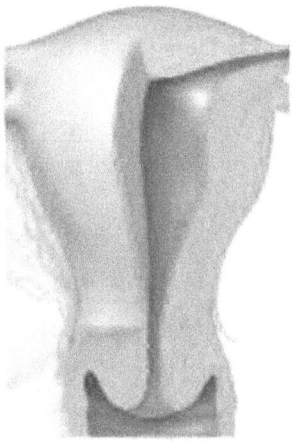

Uterine Cavity

The uterus is connected to its surrounding structures by a series of ligaments and connective tissue.

The pelvic peritoneum is attached to the body and the cervix as the broad ligament, reflecting onto the bladder, and attaches the uterus to the lateral pelvic side walls.

Within the broad base of the broad ligament, between its anterior and posterior laminae, connective tissue strands associated with the uterine and vaginal vessels help to support the uterus and vagina; together, these strands are referred to as the cardinal ligament.

Rectouterine ligaments, lying within peritoneal folds, stretch posteriorly from the cervix to reach the sacrum.

The round ligaments of the uterus are much denser structures and connect the uterus to the anterolateral abdominal wall at the deep inguinal ring; they lie within the anterior lamina of the broad ligament.

Within the round ligament is the artery of Sampson, a small artery that must be ligated during hysterectomy.

The vasculature of the uterus is derived from the uterine arteries and veins.

The uterine vessels arise from the anterior division of the internal iliac, and branches of the uterine artery anastomose with the ovarian artery along the uterine tube.

Lymphatic drainage is primarily to the lateral aortic, pelvic, and iliac nodes that surround the iliac vessels.

The nerve supply is attained through

– The sympathetic nervous system (by way of the hypogastric and ovarian plexuses) and

– The parasympathetic nervous system (by way of the pelvic splanchnic nerves from the second through fourth sacral nerves).

Microscopic Anatomy

The uterine corpus has 3 layers, from innermost to outermost:

(1) The endometrium is composed of of 2 layers:

– The basal layer lies next to the myometrium and contains stem cells, blood vessels and glands; it builds the functional layer in response to changing levels of estrogens and progesterone produced in the ovary and secreted into the blood stream.

– The functional layer contains blood vessels and glands.

(2) The myometrium is composed of 3 layers of smooth muscle.

(3) The serosa is a continuation of the visceral peritoneum.

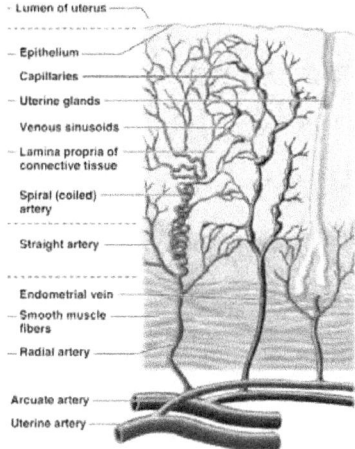

Endometrium

Functional Anatomy

It contains and nourishes the embryo and fetus from the time the fertilized egg is implanted to the time of birth of the fetus.

ENDOMETRIAL CYCLE

Proliferative Phase

The preovulatory follicular phase begins with menses; FSH and LH are released with each GnRH pulse.

Inhibin secretion is low so that FSH, which began to rise late in the luteal phase of the prior cycle, continues to rise.

At the same time, LH levels start to rise slowly.

Several secondary follicles of different sizes are recruited, and they secrete increasing amounts of estrogen and inhibin.

Estrogen and IGF-I increase the sensitivity of the follicle to FSH, while inhibin blunts the pituitary FSH response to GnRH leading to a decrease in plasma FSH.

The follicle most sensitive to FSH continues to develop and becomes the dominant follicle.

Less developed, that is, less sensitive, follicles undergo degeneration (atresia) because of insufficient FSH.

Estrogen decreases the amplitude of GnRH pulses, as well as increases pituitary sensitivity to GnRH.

Estrogen causes proliferation and vascularization of the endometrium, and increases myometrial contractility.

Estrogen also causes the cervical mucus to become clear and thin.

Secretory Phase

When plasma estradiol exceeds 150-200 pg/mL for 36 hours, GnRH triggers a large surge of LH and a small surge of FSH.

The FSH surge recruits new follicles for the next cycle; the LH surge triggers ovulation and luteinization of follicular cells.

The corpus luteum then synthesizes increasing amounts of progesterone, estradiol, and inhibin.

FSH and LH are low, but they maintain the corpus luteum.

Progesterone decreases the frequency of GnRH pulses resulting in a decrease in the frequency of LH pulses.

The LH pulse amplitude increases, however, so that plasma LH remains unchanged.

The post-ovulatory rise in progesterone appears to be responsible for the rise in basal body temperature.

Progesterone decreases myometrial excitability and increases endometrial secretory activity.

The luteal phase has a more constant length than the follicular phase.

Menstrual Phase

If implantation of the blastocyst occurs, the lifespan of the corpus luteum is prolonged by hCG, which is produced by the developing embryo.

If implantation does not occur, the corpus luteum regresses.

Luteal regression begins 14-15 days after ovulation, and progesterone levels decrease to follicular phase levels.

The endometrial lining undergoes ischemic necrosis followed by menses, which is desquamation and bleeding.

Menstruation lasts 3-5 days, and on average, 35 ml of blood + 35 ml serous fluid are lost.

One day before menstruation, when the inhibin levels are low, FSH begins to rise - the proliferative phase is again initiated.

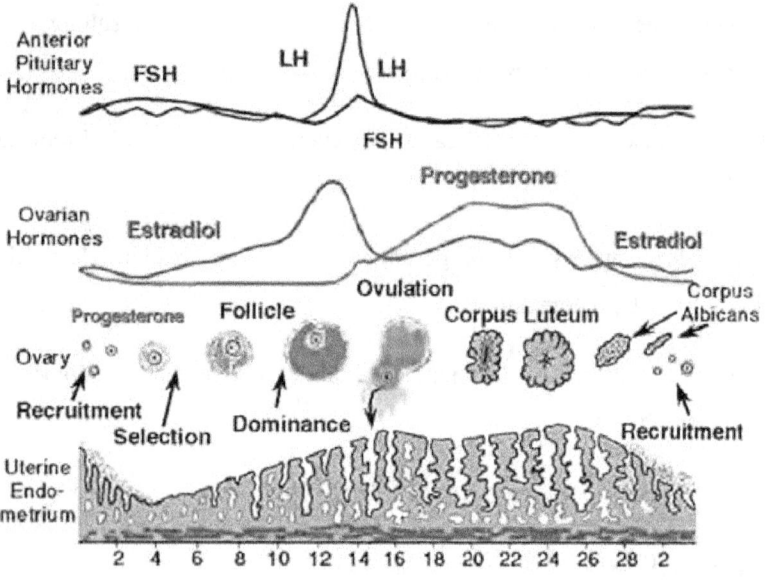

Menstrual Cycle

IMPLANTATION

Approximately seven days after fertilization, the blastocyst bursts from the zona pellucida (hatching) and implants in the wall of the uterus.

Implantation requires prior conditioning of the endometrium by progesterone, which causes the stromal cells to swell and accumulate glycogen, lipids and protein.

The presence of hCG from the blastocyst stimulates the corpus luteum of the maternal ovary to secrete progesterone.

The blastocyst attaches to the uterine fundus at the embryonic pole.

Trophoblast cells then invade through the endometrial epithelium into the endometrial stroma aided by proteases.

Stromal cells decidualize; a process by which they enlarge and become transcriptionally active, and surround the blastocyst.

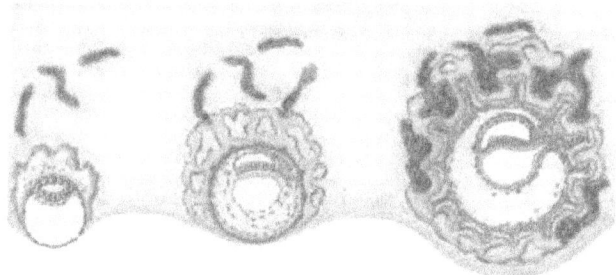

Implantation

EMBRYO DEVELOPMENT

The zygote is kept in the fallopian tube for about three days by the spastic contractions of the estrogen-dominated isthmus; as progesterone increases, muscle tone decreases.

In the fallopian tube, the zygote undergoes cleavage division (1-cell to 8-cell), compaction and blastocyst formation.

The inner cell mass becomes the fetus and the outer cells become the placenta and fetal membranes.

Peristalsis moves the fertilized oocyte through the tubal isthmus and into the uterus for implantation.

Approximately seven days after fertilization, the blastocyst bursts from the zona pellucida, which is called hatching, and implants in the wall of the uterus, which is called nidation.

Implantation requires prior conditioning of the endometrium by progesterone, which causes the stromal cells to swell and accumulate glycogen, lipids and protein.

The presence of hCG from the blastocyst stimulates the corpus luteum of the maternal ovary to secrete progesterone.

The blastocyst attaches to the wall of the uterine fundus at the embryonic pole.

Trophoblast cells then invade through the endometrial epithelium into the endometrial stroma aided by proteases.

Stromal cells decidualize; a process by which they enlarge and become transcriptionally active, and surround the blastocyst.

Within 11 days of fertilization, the trophoblast forms two layers, the cytotrophoblast and the syncytiotrophoblast, containing lacunae.

The placenta forms a barrier to permit exchange of nutrients, gases and wastes with only slight mixing of fetal blood with maternal blood.

Fetal blood cells can normally be found in the maternal circulation in all cases.

As the lacunae enlarge, the trophoblast forms villi, which consist of a vascularized core of cytotrophoblast covered by syncytiotrophoblast.

The trophoblast erodes the maternal spiral arteries, which then flow directly into the intervillous spaces.

The fully developed placenta consists of the following three layers of membranes:

– Amnion (inner), which is a single layer of ectodermal epithelium completely enclosing the embryo;

– Chorion (outer), which surrounds the amniotic sac and includes the villi and trophoblast; and

– The decidua of the maternal endometrium.

The uterofetoplacental circulation is established by about 6 gestational weeks and is completed by 10 weeks, connecting the maternal decidua through the chorionic villi to the fetus via the umbilical vessels.

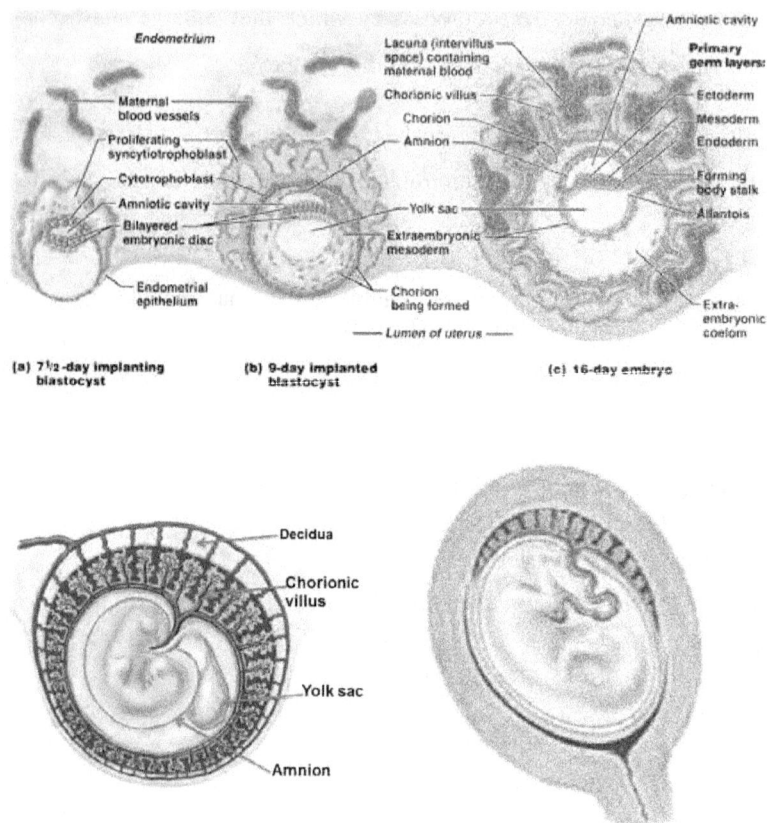

(a) 7½-day implanting blastocyst

(b) 9-day implanted blastocyst

(c) 16-day embryo

Embryo Development

UTERINE FACTORS OF INFERTILITY

The uterus is the final destination for the embryo and the place where the fetus develops until delivery.

Therefore, uterine factors may be associated with primary infertility or with pregnancy wastage and premature delivery.

Causes

Uterine factors can be congenital or acquired.

They may affect the endometrium or myometrium and are responsible for 2-5% of infertility cases.

Congenital Defects

The full spectrum of congenital/müllerian abnormalities varies from total absence of the uterus and vagina (Rokitansky-Küster-Hauser syndrome) to minor defects such as arcuate uterus and vaginal septa (transverse or longitudinal).

The most common uterine malformations observed during the past 40 years were drug induced.

From the late 1950s until the early 1970s, diethylstilbestrol (DES) was used to treat patients with a history of recurrent miscarriages.

Years later, DES was found to be responsible for inducing malformations of the uterine cervix, irregularities of the endometrial cavity (eg, T-shaped uterus), malfunction of the fallopian tubes, menstrual irregularities, and the development of clear cell carcinoma of the vagina.

In 1988, the American Fertility Society (AFS) established a new classification of müllerian anomalies.

The purpose of this classification was to gather prospective clinical information, to determine its relevance, and to generate future recommendations for patient care.

The relationship between müllerian anomalies and infertility is not entirely clear except when absolute absence of the uterus, cervix, vagina, or a combination of these occurs.

Premature delivery has been associated with cervical incompetence, unicornuate uterus associated with a blind horn, and septate uterus.

Septate uterus may also be responsible for implantation problems and first-trimester miscarriages.

Acquired Defects

Endometritis associated with a traumatic delivery, dilatation and curettage, intrauterine device, or any instrumentation of the endometrial cavity may create intrauterine adhesions or synechiae (ie, Asherman syndrome), with partial or total obliteration of the endometrial cavity.

Intrauterine and submucosal fibroids are very common, affecting 25-50% of women.

They are more common in women of African descent and can cause distortion of the cavity and compromise the blood supply.

They may also be implicated in implantation failure, early miscarriages, premature delivery, and abruptio placentae.

Investigations

Many defects can be detected during the pelvic examination.

Detection of most defects requires ancillary studies such as HSG, pelvic ultrasonography, hysterosonogram, and MRI.

Operative procedures such as laparoscopy and hysteroscopy are often necessary for confirmation of the final diagnosis.

Hysterosalpingogram (HSG)

HSG is the most frequently used diagnostic tool to evaluate the endometrial cavity and fallopian tubes.

Some have tried to displace the role of HSG in the evaluation of infertility; however, a meticulous and well-executed procedure, performed under fluoroscopy, provides accurate information about:

– Endocervical canal.

– Diameter and configuration of the internal os.

– Endometrial cavity.

– Uterine/tubal junction (cornual ostium).

– Diameter, location, and direction of the fallopian tubes.

– Status of the fimbriae.

– Spill into the endometrial cavity.

Furthermore, the HSG provides indirect evidence of pelvic adhesions and uterine, ovarian, or adnexal masses.

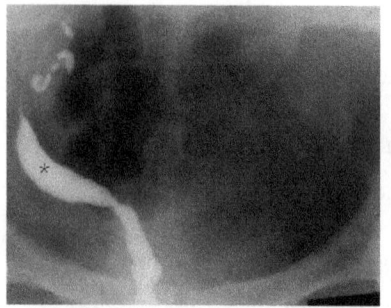

Unicornous Uterus

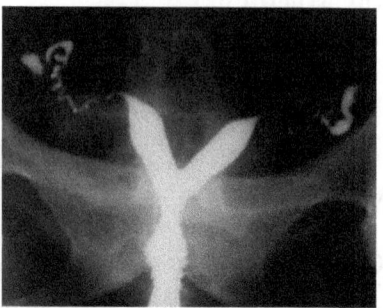

Bicornate Uterus

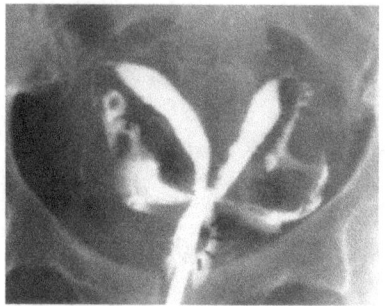

Septate Uterus

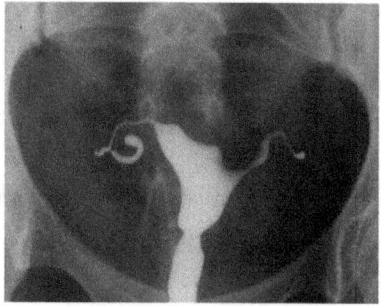

Submucous Fibroid

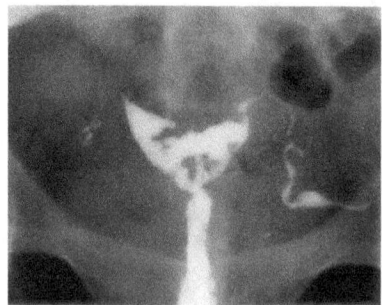

Endometrial Polyps

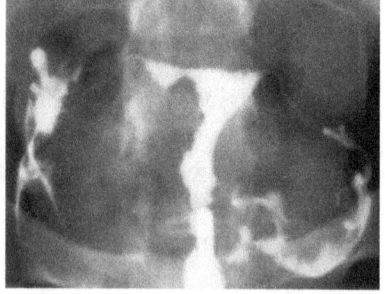

Intrauterine Adhesions

Hysterosalpingogram (HSG)

Ultrasonography

In the 1980s, pelvic ultrasonography became an important tool in the evaluation and monitoring of infertile patients, especially during ovulation induction.

Pelvic ultrasonography should be part of the routine gynecologic evaluation because it allows a more precise evaluation of the position of the uterus within the pelvis and provides more information about its size and irregularities.

Pelvic sonograms also help in the early detection of uterine fibroids, endometrial polyps, ovarian cysts, adnexal masses, and endometriomas.

Ultrasonography can also assist in the diagnosis of anovulation, polycystic ovaries, and persistent corpus luteum cysts.

Saline Infusion Sonography (SIS)

SIS provides a simple and inexpensive means by which to evaluate the uterine cavity and assess tubal patency.

It is well-tolerated by patients and can be done in the office.

Additionally, it eliminates the risks associated with the use of dye and radiation required by the HSG.

SIS has been shown to reveal a substantial percentage of infertile patients with intracavitary abnormalities and uterine anomalies.

SIS should be performed during cycle days 6-12 so that the endometrium is thin, allowing better detection of intrauterine lesions, in addition, this ensures that an undiagnosed pregnancy is not disrupted.

A breakaway speculum is placed and the cervix is cleansed with Betadine solution.

A transcervical catheter with acorn or balloon is placed.

The speculum is removed and saline is injected under ultrasonographic visualization.

Longitudinal and transverse views of the cavity are evaluated.

Finally, a small amount of air bubbles are injected to assess tubal patency.

If the patient has a history of genital tract infection or PID, antibiotics may be given before the procedure.

While the SIS can confirm tubal patency, it does not provide information about the contour of the tubes.

Thus, if a patient has a history of endometriosis or other tubal disease, an HSG would be preferred.

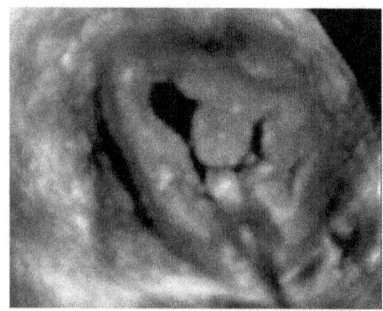   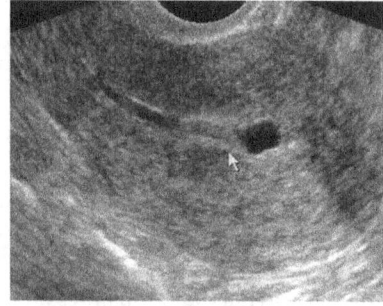

Submucous Fibroid   **Intrauterine Adhesions**

Saline Infusion Sonography (SIS)

Magnetic Resonance Imaging (MRI)

The use of MRI has increased in recent years, although it should be limited to those patients in whom a definitive diagnosis cannot be ascertained by conventional HSG, ultrasonography, and hysteroscopy.

MRI is useful for delineating complex pelvic masses and for assisting in the diagnosis of such conditions as congenital malformations related to cryptomenorrhea and absence of the cervix.

Hysteroscopy

Hysteroscopy is a method of direct visualization of endometrial cavity.

The instrument used has evolved from the historical cystoscope and is based on the same principles.

The technology has changed substantially and now uses optical devices, video camera-enhanced images, and television monitors, which allow more efficient participation and coordination of other members of the operating room team.

The use of glycine and sorbitol solutions, different from the classic Hyskon, administered under constant pressure using an automatic pump, improves imaging resolution and is less risky to the patient.

The diameter of the device has become smaller, making it more user friendly; thus, the procedure can be performed in the physician's office using local anesthesia (ie, paracervical block).

The operative hysteroscope has been designed based on the resectoscope principle.

It allows both the diagnosis and treatment of endometrial pathology.

The design of refined instruments (eg, scissors, cautery loops, lasers) facilitated the treatment of pathologies such as uterine synechiae, endometrial polyps, submucous myomas, and the removal of foreign bodies (eg, intrauterine devices).

In combination with specially designed catheters, it can be used to perform tubal cannulation.

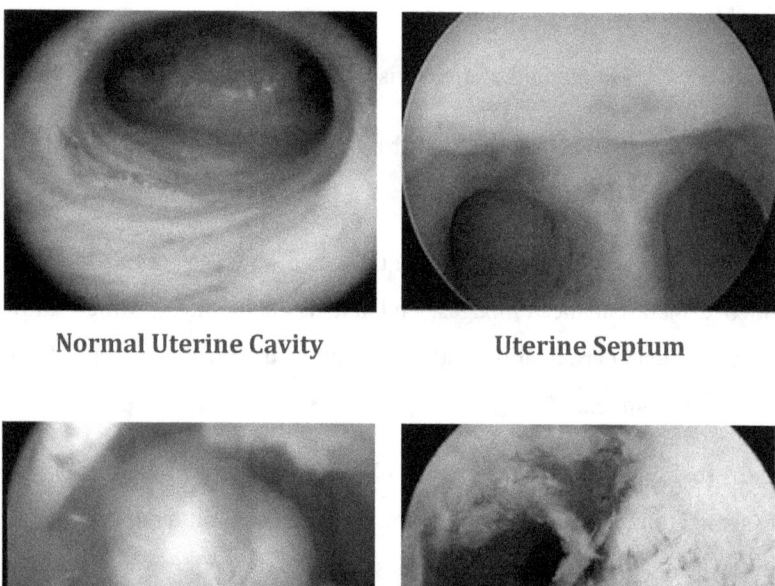

Normal Uterine Cavity   Uterine Septum

Submucous Fibroid   Intrauterine Adhesions

Hysteroscopy

Endometrial Biopsy

The endometrial lining constantly responds to the different hormonal secretions that occur during the menstrual cycle or to the exogenous administration of estrogen and progesterone.

In the 1950s, Novack and Noyes published their findings on the microscopic changes of the endometrium throughout the menstrual cycle and established the criteria for endometrial dating.

Jones first described the luteal phase dysfunction and its association with recurrent pregnancy loss.

A luteal phase dysfunction diagnosis is based on the lack of correlation between endometrial development, diagnosed using premenstrual endometrial biopsy, and the onset of the immediate menstrual cycle.

To fulfill the diagnostic criteria, more than 2 days' difference must exist between the endometrial date and the beginning of the next menstrual period.

Furthermore, the same findings should be repeated in 2 consecutive menstrual cycles.

A large, multi-center prospective study showed that out-of-phase biopsy results poorly discriminated between women from fertile and infertile couples in either the midluteal or late luteal phase.

Therefore, histological dating of the endometrium does not discriminate between women of fertile and infertile couples and should not be used in the routine evaluation of infertility.

Treatment

Until IVF became available, a patient with congenital absence of the uterus and vagina (Rokitansky-Küster-Hauser syndrome) had no chance to have a biologic child.

Today, it is feasible by using a surrogate mother or gestational carrier.

Once patients desire to have children, they proceed with stimulation of the ovaries, oocyte aspiration, and IVF, but the embryos are transferred to a gestational carrier.

The treatment of uterine malformations depends on the severity of the problem.

Fertility is not an issue for some patients affected by DES, and they remain undiagnosed until they have an abnormal Papanicolaou test result.

Those who do have fertility problems are treated according to the following guidelines:

– Chronic cervical factor of absence of mucus – IUI.

– Cervical incompetence – Cerclage.

– Damage/absence of fallopian tubes (ectopic) – IVF.

Unicornuate Uterus

A unicornuate uterus remains undetected unless fertility is compromised.

Patients with this type of uterus can have a normal term pregnancy.

Most problems are related to premature labor and pregnancy loss.

Unicornuate uterus is associated with renal abnormalities including absence of a kidney or presence of a pelvic kidney; this occurs in 15% of cases.

Thus, an intravenous pyelogram must be performed once this diagnosis is made.

Whether interventions before conception or early in pregnancy, such as resection of the rudimentary horn and prophylactic cervical cerclage, decidedly improve obstetrical outcomes is uncertain.

Women presenting with a history of this anomaly should be considered high-risk obstetrical patients.

Bicornuate Uterus

A bicornuate uterus causes only minimal problems with infertility (if any).

A bicornuate uterus can be associated with a history of recurrent miscarriages, and its repair is indicated only if other etiologies for the miscarriage have been excluded.

Arcuate Uterus

In general, an arcuate uterus does not cause infertility.

Whether it should be corrected in cases of primary infertility is controversial.

Septate Uterus

The hypothesis that a uterine septum can cause infertility is controversial.

Advising surgery in cases of primary infertility is difficult.

The avascular nature of the septum is theorized to interfere with implantation and maintenance of the embryo.

Uterine anomalies can be corrected through operative hysteroscopy under general anesthesia or conscious sedation.

Ideally, the procedure should be performed during the early follicular phase and under laparoscopic surveillance to decrease the risk of uterine perforation.

Furthermore, laparoscopy assists in the differential diagnosis between a septate and a bicornuate uterus.

A bicornuate uterus is characterized by the presence of an indentation at the fundus.

The 2 techniques are the Strassman metroplasty and the Jones metroplasty.

The Strassman metroplasty consists of performing an incision at the fundus of the uterus between both cornual areas and closing the defect with an anteroposterior suture.

Jones metroplasty consists of resecting the septum using anteroposterior wedge incision and closing the defect in the same direction.

Uterine Synechiae

Uterine synechiae are corrected using operative hysteroscopy.

The surgery is performed during the early follicular phase.

Once the synechiae have been resected, leaving an intrauterine balloon for 7 days is advisable to prevent a recurrence of adhesions.

The patient should receive prophylactic antibiotics and uterine relaxants (eg, ibuprofen) during these 7 days to prevent infection and balloon expulsion, respectively.

The patient should be prescribed high-dose estradiol (5 mg qd for 21 d) followed by medroxyprogesterone (10 mg for 10 d).

A postoperative HSG should be performed 2 months later.

In many instances, more than one hysteroscopy is required.

Endometrial Polyps

Endometrial polyps are removed through operative hysteroscopy associated with a dilatation and curettage, if necessary.

An HSG follow-up procedure is not necessary.

To prevent further polyp development associated with anovulation, the patient should have withdrawal bleeding at least every 6 weeks.

Uterine Fibroids

In general, small and asymptomatic myomas do not require treatment, but the patient should be periodically monitored.

Fibroids should be treated if they are associated with abnormal uterine bleeding or if they are thought to be the cause of infertility.

Three modalities are used to treat myomas: medical treatment, surgical treatment, and embolization.

Medical treatment is a temporary treatment, ideally used for patients who are close to menopause or who are risky surgical candidates.

However, medical treatment can be used to reduce the myoma size prior to removal. GnRH analog (eg. leuprolide acetate) causes down-regulation of the pituitary, inducing chemical menopause after injections of 3.75 mg intramuscularly every 4 weeks for a period of up to 6 months.

Disadvantages of this treatment include symptoms of menopause, osteoporosis, and recurrence of the myomas after discontinuation of the treatment.

Surgical treatment of myomas is indicated in cases of abnormal uterine bleeding, when the myoma is implicated in recurrent miscarriages or when it is thought to interfere with embryo implantation.

The 3 classes of surgical techniques are conventional laparotomy, operative laparoscopy, and operative hysteroscopy.

Laparotomy is indicated for large myomas, for submucous myomas >3 cm in diameter, or for myomas that, regardless of being submucous, have a portion of the myoma that compromises the myometrium so that a complete resection through the hysteroscopy is not feasible.

Operative laparoscopy is indicated for pedunculated and superficial intramural myomas.

This technique should be reserved for myomas with a diameter <6 cm.

Several cases have been reported of uterine rupture during pregnancy because the reconstruction of the uterus after laparoscopic myomectomy was not as good as a myomectomy performed using laparotomy.

The removal of a submucous fibroid using hysteroscopy should be limited to small fibroids (≤3 cm) with minimal compromise of the myometrium.

This is important to decrease the risk of excessive bleeding and to decrease the risk of electrolyte imbalance, water intoxication, and pulmonary edema from excessive intravasation of Hyskon, glycine, or sorbitol used during the procedure.

Uterine synechiae development is a potential complication after the hysteroscopic surgery; therefore, a postoperative HSG should be part of follow-up care.

Uterine fibroid embolization consists of catheterization of the uterine artery and the injection of microbeads of polyvinyl alcohol to selectively occlude the circulation of the fibroid.

The procedure is performed by interventional radiology and requires overnight admission for the patient.

It is not intended for patients who desire fertility.

CERVIX

The cervix is the inferior portion of the uterus, separating the body of the uterus from the vagina; its average length is 3-5 cm.

The cervix is cylindrical in shape, with an endocervical canal located in the midline, allowing passage of semen into the uterus.

The external opening into the vagina is termed the external os; and the internal opening into the endometrial cavity is termed the internal os.

The internal os is the portion of a female cervix that dilates to allow delivery of the fetus during labor.

The vasculature is supplied by descending branches of the uterine artery, which run bilaterally at the 3 o'clock and 9 o'clock position of the cervix.

Lymphatic drainage of the cervix is complex: the obturator, common iliac, internal iliac, external iliac, and visceral parametrial nodes are the main drainage points.

The nerve supply to the cervix is via the parasympathetic nervous system by way of the second through fourth sacral segments; many pain nerve fibers run alongside these parasympathetics.

Microscopic Anatomy

Most of the cervix is composed of collagenous connective tissue, smooth muscle, and mucopolysaccharide ground substance.

The endocervical canal is rich in mucous glands and is primarily columnar epithelium.

The external portion of the cervix that lies within the vagina is composed of stratified squamous epithelium.

The area surrounding the external os is termed the transformation zone, which is the transition point between squamous cells externally and columnar cells of the endocervical canal.

Functional Anatomy

The epithelial lining, of the cervix consists of tall, secretory columnar cells that respond to estradiol by increasing in height and accumulating cervical mucus rich in protein substances.

The mucus functions as a hormone-dependent barrier for sperm to enter the uterus.

At mid-cycle, when estrogen levels are high, mucus is clear, thin, and copious with high elasticity, called spinnbarkeit.

At this point, the cervical mucus is permeable to sperm and when dried, has a characteristic microscopic ferning appearance.

The mucus actually restricts sperm with poor morphology and motility; as a result, only a minority of ejaculated sperm actually enters the cervix.

In response to progesterone production after ovulation, mucus production decreases and it becomes viscous, cloudy, and impermeable to sperm.

CAPACITATION

After the ejaculation, the sperm cells go through several essential physiological changes during their time in the female genital tract before they, at the end, are able to penetrate the oocyte membrane.

The first change in this cascade is capacitation, which is physiological maturation process of the sperm cell membranes.

The sperm cells accomplish this during the ascension through the female genital tract (in contact with its secretions); the cervix may act as a site where capacitation of the sperm might start.

The changes take place via the sperm cell membrane in which it may be that receptors are made available through removal of a glycoprotein layer.

The area of the acrosomal cap is also so altered thereby that the acrosome reaction becomes possible.

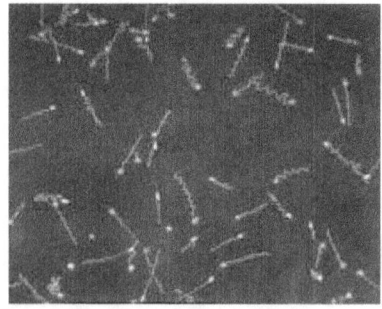 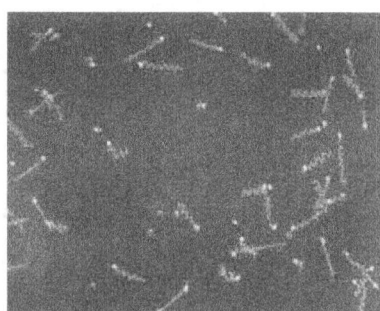

Before Capacitation   **After Capacitation**

CERVICAL FACTORS OF INFERTILITY

The uterine cervix plays a pivotal role in the transport and capacitation of the sperm after intercourse.

Cervical factors account for 5-10% of infertility.

Causes

Cervical factor infertility can be caused by stenosis or abnormalities of the mucus-sperm interaction.

Cervical mucus production and characteristics change according to the estrogen concentration during the late follicular phase.

At the beginning of the menstrual cycle, cervical mucus is scanty, viscous, and very cellular forming a netlike structure that does not allow the passage of sperm.

Mucus secretion increases during the mid follicular phase and reaches its maximum approximately 24-48 hours before ovulation.

The water and salt concentration increases, changing the physical characteristics of the mucus.

The mucus becomes thin, watery, alkaline, acellular, and elastic (spinnbarkheit) because of the increased concentration of sodium chloride, despite a fernlike pattern when the mucus is allowed to dry on a cover slide under the microscope.

At this point, the mucus organizes itself, forming multiple microchannels so the spermatozoa can travel through.

During this journey, the spermatozoa simultaneously undergo activation and capacitation.

In addition, the mucus acts as a filter for abnormal spermatozoa and cellular debris present in the semen.

Mucus secretion may be altered by hormonal changes and medications, especially drugs like CC, which decrease the production.

Hypoestrogenism may cause thickened cervical mucus, which impairs the passage of sperm.

Cervical stenosis can cause infertility by blocking the passage of sperm from the cervix to the intrauterine cavity.

Cervical stenosis can be congenital or acquired in etiology, resulting from surgical procedures, infections, hypoestrogenism, and radiation therapy.

Investigations

Cervical stenosis can be diagnosed during a speculum examination.

Complete cervical stenosis is confirmed by the inability to pass a 1-2 mm probe into the uterine cavity.

The postcoital test (PCT), also known as the Sims-Huhner test, consists of evaluating the amount of spermatozoa and its motility within the cervical mucus during the preovulatory period.

This test is no longer routinely performed in the standard infertility workup because it has been shown to have limited diagnostic potential.

Furthermore, cervical factor infertility is easily addressed by IUI.

Treatment

Chronic cervicitis may be treated with antibiotics.

Reduced secretion of cervical mucus due to destruction of the endocervical glands by previous cervical conization, freezing, or laser vaporization responds poorly to low-dose estrogen therapy.

The easiest and most successful treatment is IUI.

Similar treatments apply when oligospermia, hypospermia, and ejaculatory disorders such as impotence, hypospadias, or retrograde ejaculation are present.

Artificial insemination can be performed by depositing the sperm at the cervical level (cervical insemination) or inside the endometrial cavity (IUI).

Cervical insemination has almost been abandoned because of its low success.

It has been relegated only to cases in which the sperm count is normal, or if the sample has elevated white cells.

For IUI, IVF, and ICSI procedures, the removal of certain components of the ejaculate (ie, seminal fluid, excess cellular debris, leukocytes, morphologically abnormal sperm) with the retention of the motile fraction of sperm is desirable.

For most specimens, the greatest recovery of the motile portion results from separation via centrifugal filtration through a discontinuous density gradient system.

However, for certain very poor specimens with low original concentrations of motile sperm, the use of the gradient system results in such a negligible recovery as to render it useless.

A small number of specimens have acceptable original concentrations of motile sperm but poor recoveries with the gradient system.

These specimens benefit most from layering a washed pellet of sperm with nutrient media and allowing the motile fraction to swim up into the media before being separated.

IUI is performed during a natural cycle or after ovulation induction with CC or gonadotropins.

The procedure is performed 30-34 hours after the spontaneous LH surge or 36 hours after the administration of 10,000 IU of hCG.

The sperm is delivered into the endometrial cavity using an IUI catheter.

After injection of the sperm, the patient remains in the recumbent position for 10-15 minutes.

The average pregnancy rate achieved after a natural-cycle IUI is 8%; increases to 10-12% after CC ovulation induction and to 12-15% per cycle after hMG/hCG ovulation induction; 85% of the successful pregnancies are achieved within the first 4 cycles of IUI.

REFERENCES

– Al-Azemi M, Killick SR, Duffy S, et al. Multi-marker assessment of ovarian reserve predicts oocyte yield after ovulation induction. Hum Reprod. 2011; 26: 414-22.

– American Society for Reproductive Medicine. Use of clomiphene citrate in women. ASRM Committee Opinion. Fertil Steril. 2006; 86: S187-93.

– American Society for Reproductive Medicine. Use of exogenous gonadotropins in anovulatory women. ASRM Technical Bulletin. Fertil Steril. 2008; 90: S7-12.

– American Society for Reproductive Medicine. Gonadotropin preparations: past, present, and future perspectives. ASRM Educational Bulletin. Fertil Steril. 2008; 90: S13-20.

– Badawy A, Mosbah A, Tharwat A, et al. Extended letrozole therapy for ovulation induction in clomiphene-resistant women with polycystic ovary syndrome: a novel protocol. Fertil Steril. 2009; 92: 236-9.

– Barnhart K, Dunsmoor-Su R, Coutifaris C. Effect of endometriosis on in vitro fertilization. Fertil Steril. 2002: 77; 1148-55.

– Bedaiwy MA, Mousa NA, Esfandiari N, et al. Follicular phase dynamics with combined aromatase inhibitor and follicle stimulating hormone treatment. J Clin Endocrinol Metab. 2007; 92: 825-33.

– Berin I, Stein DE, Keltz MD. A comparison of gonadotropin-releasing hormone (GnRH) antagonist and GnRH agonist flare protocols for poor responders undergoing in vitro fertilization. Fertil Steril. 2010; 93: 360-3.

– Braun DP, Dmowski WP. Endometriosis: abnormal endometrium and dysfunctional immune response. Curr Opin Obstet Gynecol. 1998; 10: 365-9.

– Broekmans FJ, Kwee J, Hendriks DJ, et al. A systematic review of tests predicting ovarian reserve and IVF outcome. Hum Reprod Update. 2006; 12: 685-718.

– Buckingham KL, Chamley LW. A critical assessment of the role of antiphospholipid antibodies in infertility. J Reprod Immunol. 2009: 80; 132-45.

– Buyalos RP, Daneshmand S, Brzechffa PR. Basal estradiol and follicle-stimulating hormone predict fecundity in women of advanced reproductive age undergoing ovulation induction therapy. Fertil Steril. 1997; 68: 272-7.

– Caburet S, Arboleda VA, Llano E, et al. Mutant Cohesin in Premature Ovarian Failure. N Engl J Med. 2014; 370: 943-9.

– Casper RF, Mitwally MF. Review: aromatase inhibitors for ovulation induction. J Clin Endocrinol Metab. 2006; 91: 760-71.

– Centers for Disease Control and Prevention, American Society for Reproductive Medicine, Society for Assisted Reproductive Technology. 2006 Assisted Reproductive Technology Success Rates: National Summary and Fertility Clinic Reports, Atlanta: U.S. Department of Health and Human Services, Centers for Disease Control and Prevention; 2008.

– Chamley LW, Clarke GN. Antisperm antibodies and conception. Semin Immunopathol. 2007: 29; 169-84.

– Chung KW. Gross Anatomy. 4th ed. Philadelphia: Lippincott Williams & Wilkins; 2000.

– Cline AM, Kutteh WH. Is there a role of autoimmunity in implantation failure after in-vitro fertilization? Curr Opin Obstet Gynecol. 2009: 21; 291-5.

– Coutifaris C, Myers ER, Guzick DS, et al. Histological dating of timed endometrial biopsy tissue is not related to fertility status. Fertil Steril. 2004; 82: 1264-72.

– Coviello AD, Legro RS, Dunaif A. Adolescent girls with polycystic ovary syndrome have an increased risk of the metabolic syndrome associated with increasing androgen levels independent of obesity and insulin resistance. J Clin Endocrinol Metab. 2006; 92: 492-7.

– Daya S. Updated meta-analysis of recombinant follicle-stimulating hormone (FSH) versus urinary FSH for ovarian stimulation in assisted reproduction. Fertil Steril. 2002; 77: 711-4.

– Dechanet C, Anahory T, Mathieu Daude JC, et al. Effects of cigarette smoking on reproduction. Hum Reprod Update. 2011; 17: 76-95.

– Dickey RP, Holtkamp DE. Development, pharmacology, and clinical experience with clomiphene citrate. Hum Reprod Update. 1996; 2: 483-506.

– Donckers J, Evers JL, Land JA. The long-term outcome of 946 consecutive couples visiting a fertility clinic in 2001-2003. Fertil Steril. 2011; 96: 160-4.

– Dovey S, Sneeringer RM, Penzias AS. Clomiphene citrate and intrauterine insemination: analysis of more than 4100 cycles. Fertil Steril. 2008; 90: 2281-6.

– Drake RL, Vogl AW, Mitchell AWM. Gray's Anatomy for Student's. 2nd ed. Philadelphia: Churchill Livingstone Elsevier; 2010.

– Eftekhari N, Mohammadalizadeh S. Pregnancy rate following bromocriptine treatment in infertile women with galactorrhea. Gynecol Endocrinol. 2009; 25: 122-4.

– Ehrmann DA, Barnes RB, Rosenfeld RL, et al. Prevalence of impaired glucose tolerance and diabetes in women with polycystic ovary syndrome. Diabetes Care. 1999; 22: 141-6.

– Engmann L, DiLuigi A, Schmidt D, et al. The use of gonadotropin-releasing hormone (GnRH) agonist to induce oocyte maturation after cotreatment with GnRH antagonist in high-risk patients undergoing in vitro fertilization prevents the risk of ovarian hyperstimulation syndrome: a prospective randomized controlled study. Fertil Steril. 2008; 89: 84-91.

– Forman R, Gill S, Moretti M, et al. Fetal safety of letrozole and clomiphene citrate for ovulation induction. J Obstet Gynaecol Can. 2007; 29: 668-71.

– García-Ulloa AC, Arrieta O. Tubal occlusion causing infertility due to an excessive inflammatory response in patients with predisposition for keloid formation. Med. Hypotheses 2005; 65: 908–14.

– Gillen-water JY, Grayhack JT, Howards SS, et al. Adult and pediatric urology. 4th ed. London: Lippincott. Williams & Wilkins; 2002.

– Gray H. Anatomy, Descriptive and Surgical. The Unabridged Gray's Anatomy. Philadelphia: Running Press; 1999.

– Hoover RN, Hyer M, Pfeiffer RM, et al. Adverse health outcomes in women exposed in utero to diethylstilbestrol. N Engl J Med. 2011; 365: 1304-14.

– Huang H, Lv C, Zhao Y, et al. Mutant ZP1 in Familial Infertility. N Engl J Med. 2014; 370: 1220-6.

– Imani B, Eijkemans MJ, te Velde ER, et al. A nomogram to predict the probability of live birth after clomiphene citrate induction of ovulation in normogonadotropic oligoamenorrheic infertility. Fertil Steril. 2002; 77: 91-7.

– Kallio S, Aittomäki K, Piltonen T, et al. Anti-Mullerian hormone as a predictor of follicular reserve in ovarian insufficiency: special emphasis on FSH-resistant ovaries. Hum Reprod. 2012; 27: 854-60.

– Kashyap S, Parker K, Cedars MI, et al. Ovarian hyperstimulation syndrome prevention strategies: reducing the human chorionic gonadotropin trigger dose. Semin Reprod Med. 2010; 28: 475-85.

– Katz VL, Lentz GM, Lobo RA, et al. Comprehensive Gynecology. 5th ed. Philadelphia: Mosby Elsevier; 2007.

– Kim MD, Kim NK, Kim HJ, et al. Pregnancy following uterine artery embolization with polyvinyl alcohol particles for patients with uterine fibroid or adenomyosis. Cardiovasc Intervent Radiol. 2005; 28: 611-5.

– Knochenhauer ES, Key TJ, Kahsar-Miller M, et al. Prevalence of the polycystic ovary syndrome in unselected black and white women of the southeastern United States: a prospective study. J Clin Endocrinol Metab. 1998; 83: 3078-82.

– Kolodziejczyk B, Duleba AJ, Spaczynski RZ, et al. Metformin therapy decreases hyperandrogenism and hyperinsulinemia in women with polycystic ovary syndrome. Fertil Steril. 2000; 73: 1149-54.

– Koninckx PR, Kennedy SH, Barlow DH. Endometriotic disease: the role of peritoneal fluid. Hum Reprod Update. 1998; 4: 741-51.

– Koning AM, Kuchenbecker WK, Groen H, et al. Economic consequences of overweight and obesity in infertility: a framework for evaluating the costs and outcomes of fertility care. Hum Reprod Update. 2010; 16: 246-54.

– Kosugi Y, Elias S, Malinak LR, et al. Increased heterogeneity of chromosome 17 aneuploidy in endometriosis. Am J Obstet Gynecol. 1999; 180: 792-7.

– Laughlin GA, Dominguez CE, Yen SS. Nutritional and endocrine-metabolic aberrations in women with functional hypothalamic amenorrhea. J Clin Endocrinol Metab. 1998; 83: 25-32.

– Legro RS, Barnhart HX, Schlaff WD, et al. Cooperative Multicenter Reproductive Medicine Network. Clomiphene, metformin, or both for infertility in the polycystic ovary syndrome. N Engl J Med. 2007; 356: 551-66.

– Lord JM, Flight IH, Norman RJ. Metformin in polycystic ovary syndrome: systematic review and meta-analysis. BMJ. 2003; 327: 951-3.

– Loukas M, Colburn GL, Abrahams P, et al. Gray's Anatomy Review. Philadelphia: Churchill Livingstone Elsevier; 2010.

– Macklon D, Fauser C. Medical approaches to ovarian stimulation for infertility. In: Jerome F. Strauss I, Robert L. Barbieri M, eds. Yen & Jaffe's Reproductive Endocrinology, 6th Edition Vol. 28. Philadelphia: Saunders, 2009: 698-708.

– Magos A. Hysteroscopic treatment of Asherman's syndrome. Reprod Biomed Online. 2002; 4: S46-51.

– Marcus MD, Loucks TL, Berga SL Psychological correlates of functional hypothalamic amenorrhea. Fertil Steril. 2001; 76: 310-6.

– Mulders AGMGJ, Laven JSE, Eijkemans MJC, et al. Patient predictors for outcome of gonadotrophin ovulation induction in women with normogonadotrophic anovulatory infertility: a meta-analysis. Hum Reprod Update. 2003; 9: 429-49.

– Neill J. Knobil and Neill's Physiology of Reproduction. 3rd ed. St. Louis, MO: Elsevier; 2006.

– Ovalle WK, Nahirney PC. Netter's Eseential Histology. Philadelphia: Sauders Elsevier; 2007.

– Palomba S, Orio F, Falbo A, et al. Clomiphene citrate versus metformin as first-line approach for the treatment of anovulation in infertile patients with polycystic ovary syndrome. J Clin Endocrinol Metab. 2007; 92: 3498-503.

– Practice Committee of the American Society for Reproductive Medicine. Endometriosis and Infertility. Fertil Steril. 2006; 86: S156-60.

– Practice Committee of the American Society for Reproductive Medicine. Optimal evaluation of the infertile female. Fertil Steril. 2006; 86: S264-7.

– Practice Committee of American Society for Reproductive Medicine in collaboration with Society for Reproductive Endocrinology and Infertility. Optimizing natural fertility. Fertil Steril. 2008; 90: S1-6.

– Practice Committee of the American Society for Reproductive Medicine. Current Evaluation of amenorrhea. Fertil Steril. 2008; 90: S219-25.

– Proctor JA, Haney AF. Recurrent first trimester pregnancy loss is associated with uterine septum but not with bicornuate uterus. Fertil Steril. 2003; 80: 1212-5.

– Raga F, Bauset C, Remohi J, et al. Reproductive impact of congenital Müllerian anomalies. Hum Reprod. 1997; 12: 2277-81.

– Reichman D, Laufer MR, Robinson BK. Pregnancy outcomes in unicornuate uteri: a review. Fertil Steril. 2009; 91: 1886-94.

– Reindollar RH, Regan MM, Neumann PJ, et al. A randomized clinical trial to evaluate optimal treatment for unexplained infertility: the fast track and standard treatment (FASTT) trial. Fertil Steril. 2010; 94: 888-99.

– Rosendahl M, Andersen C, La Cour Freiesleben N, et al. Dynamics and mechanisms of chemotherapy-induced ovarian follicular depletion in women of fertile age. Fertil Steril. 2010; 94: 156-66.

– Rotterdam ESHRE/ASRM-Sponsored PCOS Consensus Workshop Group. Revised 2003 consensus on diagnostic criteria and long-term health risks related to polycystic ovary syndrome. Fertil Steril. 2004; 81: 19-25.

– Sadler T.W. Langman's Medical Embryology. 11th ed. Baltimore, Maryland: Lippincott Williams & Wilkins; 2010.

– Seow k, Juan C, Hwang I, et al. Laparoscopic surgery in polycystic ovary syndrome: reproductive and metabolic effects. Semin Reprod Med. 2008; 26: 101-11.

– Shin JC, Ross HL, Elias S, et al. Detection of chromosomal aneuploidy in endometriosis by multi-color fluorescence in situ hybridization (FISH). Hum Genet. 1997; 100: 401-6.

– Shuiqing M, Xuming B, Jinghe L. Pregnancy and its outcome in women with malformed uterus. Chin Med Sci J. 2002; 17: 242-5.

– Sloboda DM, Hickey M, Hart R. "Reproduction in females: the role of the early life environment". Hum Reprod Update. 2010; 17: 210-27.

– Smith LP, Hacker MR, Alper MM. Patients with severe ovarian hyperstimulation syndrome can be managed safely with aggressive outpatient transvaginal paracentesis. Fertil Steril. 2009; 92: 1953-9.

– Speroff L, Fritz M, eds. Clinical Gynecologic Endocrinology and Infertility, 7th edition. Philadelphia: Lippincot, Williams & Wilkins, 2005.

– Standring S. Gray's Anatomy. 40th ed. Edinburgh: Elsevier Churchill Livingstone; 2008.

– Sultan C, Biason-Lauber A, Philibert P. Mayer-Rokitansky-Kuster-Hauser syndrome: recent clinical and genetic findings. Gynecol Endocrinol. 2009; 25: 8-11.

– Sun W, Stegmann BJ, Henne M, et al. A new approach to ovarian reserve testing. Fertil Steril. 2008; 90: 2196-202.

– Ten Broek RPG, Kok-Krant N, Bakkum EA, et al. Different surgical techniques to reduce post-operative adhesion formation: A systematic review and meta-analysis. Hum Reprod Update. 2012; 19: 12-25.

– The Evian Annual Reproduction (EVAR) Workshop Group 2010; Fauser BCJM, Diedrich K, Bouchard P, et al. Contemporary genetic technologies and female reproduction. Hum Reprod Update. 2011; 17: 829-47.

– Thessaloniki ESHRE/ASRM – Sponsored PCOS Consensus Workshop Group. Consensus on infertility treatment related to polycystic ovary syndrome. Human Reprod. 2008; 23: 462-77.

– Tulandi T, Martin J, Al-Fadhli R, et al. Congenital malformations among 911 newborns conceived after infertility treatment with letrozole or clomiphene citrate. Fertil Steril. 2006; 85: 1761-5.

– Tur-Kaspa I, Gal M, Hartman M, et al. A prospective evaluation of uterine abnormalities by saline infusion sonohysterography in 1,009 women with infertility or abnormal uterine bleeding. Fertil Steril. 2006; 86: 1731-5.

– Vercellini P, Trespidi L, De Giorgi O, et al. Endometriosis and pelvic pain: relation to disease stage and localization. Fertil Steril. 1996; 65: 299-304.

– Wang J, Zhang W, Jiang H, et al. Mutations inHFM1in Recessive Primary Ovarian Insufficiency. N Engl J Med. 2014; 370: 972-4.

– Warren MP, Voussoughian F, Geer EB, et al. Functional hypothalamic amenorrhea: hypoleptinemia and disordered eating. J Clin Endocrinol Metab. 1999; 84: 873-7.

– Wein AJ. Campbell-Walsh Urology. 9th ed. Philadelphia: Saunders Elsevier; 2007.

– Whelan JG 3rd, Vlahos NF. The ovarian hyperstimulation syndrome. Fertil Steril. 2000; 73: 883-96.

– Wild S, Pierpoint T, McKeigue P, et al. Cardiovascular disease in women with polycystic ovary syndrome at long-term follow-up: a retrospective cohort study. Clin Endocrinol (Oxf). 2000; 52: 595-600.

– World Health Organization. WHO Laboratory Manual for the Examination and Processing of Human Semen. 5th Edition. Geneva, Switzerland: WHO; 2010.

www.ingramcontent.com/pod-product-compliance
Lightning Source LLC
Chambersburg PA
CBHW060347190526
45169CB00002B/513